Testimonials

"You have helped to further open the blossom of the yoga flower." —Kathy B., Denver, Colorado, 2012

"Marta's yoga teacher training course was the perfect fit for me. In a short amount of time we covered a vast amount of material and improved my confidence as a teacher." —Angela C., Castle Rock, Colorado, 2012

"Marta, your yoga TT has changed my yoga teaching, and I feel I am a real teacher now." —Terry C., Torrington, Wyoming, 2011

TWO HUNDRED HOUR YOGA TEACHER TRAINING MANUAL

A GUIDE TO THE FUNDAMENTALS OF YOGA

MARTA BERRY

BALBOA.
PRESS

A DIVISION OF HAY HOUSE

Balboa Press books may be ordered through booksellers or by contacting:

Balboa Press
A Division of Hay House
1663 Liberty Drive
Bloomington, IN 47403
www.balboapress.com
1 (877) 407-4847

Because of the dynamic nature of the Internet, any web addresses or links contained in this book may have changed since publication and may no longer be valid. The views expressed in this work are solely those of the author and do not necessarily reflect the views of the publisher, and the publisher hereby disclaims any responsibility for them.

The author of this book does not dispense medical advice or prescribe the use of any technique as a form of treatment for physical, emotional, or medical problems without the advice of a physician, either directly or indirectly. The intent of the author is only to offer information of a general nature to help you in your quest for emotional and spiritual well-being. In the event you use any of the information in this book for yourself, which is your constitutional right, the author and the publisher assume no responsibility for your actions.

Any people depicted in stock imagery provided by Thinkstock are models, and such images are being used for illustrative purposes only. Certain stock imagery © Thinkstock.

Print information available on the last page.

ISBN: 978-1-5043-7136-0 (sc)
ISBN: 978-1-5043-7137-7 (hc)
ISBN: 978-1-5043-7151-3 (e)

Library of Congress Control Number: 2016920719

Balboa Press rev. date: 12/19/2016

Contents

Introduction..ix
Acknowledgments xi
Meet the Author...xiii
Yoga Today...xv
References and Sources..xvii
Glossary of Asana...xix

Chapter 1   Methodology of Teaching Yoga....................1
- • Capture the Energy Level of the Student
- • Technique
- • Be in Service
- • Communication
- • Contact
- • Voice
- • Adjustment
- • Making Adjustments
- • Alignment
- • Some Other Tips
- • Distractions and Obstacles
- • Benefits
- • Suggestions and Advice for the Study of Yoga
- • Injuries
- • Bandhas
- • Class Sequence
- • Vinyasa Format
- • Description—A Classic Yoga Session
- • Sharing and Unity
- • Pranayama
- • History, Paths and Styles of Yoga
- • Yoga History
- • Four Paths of Yoga: Karma, Bhakti, Jnana, and Raja

- Different Styles of Yoga
- Ashtanga (Pattajabhi Jois)
- Final Relaxation: Guided Savasana
- Yoga and Pregnancy
- Basic Asana for Pregnancy
- Yoga Benefits for Pregnancy
- Yoga Seniors—Yoga on the Chair
- Yoga for Children
- Warrior Song (with Asana)
- Song for Sun Salutation A
- Song for Sun Salutation B
- Teach How to Breathe through Questions
- Emotional Control (an example)
- Show Faces of Sadness, Madness, and So Forth
- Remember That They Are Children

Chapter 2   Philosophy of Yoga...47
- The Eight Limbs of Yoga
- The First and Second Limbs
- Yama
- Asana
- Pranayama
- Pratyahara
- Dharana
- Dhyana
- Samadhi
- Bhakti Yoga, Mantras, Hindu Gods
- Mantra (Man, "to think"; Tra, "liberation from Samsara")
- The Two Forms of Mantra
- What Is Mala, and What Is Japa?
- Popular Forms of God in Hindu Philosophy
- Yoga Sutras
- Legend of the Birth of Patanjali

- Atman: Soul
- Meditation
- Meditation 1: Interiorizing the Mind
- Deepening Consciousness
- Gong
- Meditation 2: To Heal and Transform
- Gong
- Meditation 3: Happiness, Discovering Your Heart
- Gong
- Meditation 4: Erasing the Past
- Meditation 5: Sensation in the Body
- Gong

Chapter 3 Physical and Energetic Anatomy 77
- Muladhara
- First Chakra
- Swadhistana
- Second Chakra
- Manipura
- Third Chakra
- Anahata
- Fourth Chakra
- Vishuddha
- Fifth Chakra
- Ajna
- Sixth Chakra
- Sahasrara
- Seventh Chakra
- The Detox Path
- Shapes of the Spine
- Anatomy of the Shoulders and Cervical Spine

Chapter 4   Warm-Up 117
Chapter 5   Surya Namaskar A and B.. 119
Chapter 6   Beginner Asana.. 133
Chapter 7   Intermediate Asana 159
Chapter 8   Advanced Asana 189

Introduction

Yoga is an art, yoga is life, and yoga is the art of being alive and living the dream you desire, the dream you create.

When I first started practicing yoga about seventeen years ago, I was expecting my first daughter. I knew I needed some kind of exercise and movement, and I started my practice from scratch, following the instructions of a book called *Yoga for Pregnancy*. My life started to change for the better; I felt right away that I had found a path to follow for the rest of my life.

Some years have passed. I became a teacher of yoga and then a teacher of teachers of yoga. I have taught students to be teachers in Europe, the United States, and the Caribbean; I also led a yoga adventure to Manchu Pichu in Peru. Today I decided to publish my yoga manual to help all young students of yoga, to inspire them to follow this path, to encourage them to become teachers of yoga, to fulfill their dreams, and to empower them in their journey.

Yoga is the practice we all need if we want to strengthen the roots of our souls, bodies, and minds so we can make this life the best one we can live.

I wrote the first edition of this manual back in 2009 and made improving edits, both adding and subtracting, each time I taught a class. With the class of 2014, I decided to open my work to a larger audience of teachers and students; I decided to publish the manuals outside of their use as texts for the Marta Berry Yoga Teacher Training School. Today I want to extend the desire to spread the word to the world, to the many students who can benefit and learn the process of becoming a genuine yoga instructor; and to find success in their journeys, helping others to move properly and breathe with ease and meaning.

In this book you learn all the principles necessary for you to embark on the journey of teaching yoga. The more you learn, the better teacher you will be; you will recognize the nuances, hints, and suggestions to keep communication with others inspirational.

Remember that in the path of yoga, there is no "bad" or "wrong." We are all the same, and at the same time, we are all different. Each individual and group class is unique. Your eyes, as a teacher, need to open to see how the manifestation of each body, mind, and spirit speaks.

In this manual, master the knowledge of what to learn before you start teaching, including the following:

- Chakras and asana Sanskrit
- What is yoga? History through time.
- Paths and styles of yoga
- Structure of a vinyasa class
- Alignment of the body
- Becoming a teacher—important aspects of a teacher
- Yoga sutras: what does the Sutra 2 of Book 1 say?
- The limbs of yoga
- Hindu deities
- Understanding of pranayama
- Energetic anatomy, bandhas, nadis, kundalini, and qualities of nature
- Mantra, Japa, and Mala
- Understanding the meaning of Gayatri Mantra

The concepts you learn in this book will amplify the presence of knowledge in your classes, clarify some of the purposes of the practices, and help to create classes with diversity and variations.

Teaching yoga is fun and real; you are on your mat, and that is all that matters—not much and a lot. When you remember that all you have is your mat and your breath, the perspective of your life is transformed.

In yoga we believe in transformation from the inside out. That opens the heart to approach life with a deep sense of being alive.

Namaste,
Marta Berry

Acknowledgments

I dedicate this book to each person I have been privileged to have in my classes. This includes the diverse towns, cities, and countries where I have had the opportunity to teach—from Spain (Menorca, Barcelona, Madrid, and Valencia); to the Island of Roatan in Honduras, Central America; to Peru in South America; and of course to the greater USA (Miami. Florida; Denver, Colorado; Los Angeles and San Francisco in California; and the city of Gillette and the numerous small communities in the state of Wyoming, where students have welcomed me). I do remember all of you kindly. Thank you for your support. Without you I would never be who I am.

In addition, I need to mention my two daughters, Cheyenne Maryjoan and Julieta Alexandra, for being such great kids and unconditionally supporting me in every step of this journey. Thanks to you, girls, I became a mother and have developed most of my personality. Thank you for believing in me.

Back in Barcelona, I have an extraordinary and humongous number of family and friends. Special thanks to my sister, Cristina Guillen, for her constant support in my whole life; and to all the vineyards in Alta Alella, for all the success their efforts bring in my whole life. Today I celebrate with them.

For my husband, Paul Berry, thank you, for your continuous love and support.

Thank you to all practitioners of yoga and life. This is our school!

Namaste,
Marta Berry

Meet the Author

Marta Berry, originally from Barcelona, Spain, became a yoga instructor in 2005 under the guidance of Rosella Rossi in Asheville, North Carolina.

An avid traveler, Marta has brought her yoga teachings to many cities of the world. Her passion for yoga practice brought her to develop and create a yoga school in 2009. She wrote this manual to offer all the necessary and basic information to every student who needs guidance with the basics of yoga knowledge in an easy, fun, and obtainable manner before starting the new path of teaching yoga.

The experience you will receive along the path will give you the steadiness to trust your intuition. We are all great teachers, for what we learn we discover we have already known.

Marta Berry

Yoga Today

Yoga has become so popular in the world that almost everyone is doing it, and I am wondering why. It is well said that when you dedicate your time to the practice of yoga, the results appear in your physical, energetic, and mental aspects.

The physical body requires movement, exercise, and fluidity to find the great state of well-being. We know that training is forever.

The energetic body desires constant contact with the higher self to communicate with the peace and love that exist within. The mind looks for control and well-being. Yoga is a great practice for controlling the fluctuations of the mind.

In the realm of yoga, you define the connection between you and others. The physical practice of yoga will open the doors to a stronger and more efficient you; the energetic part of yoga takes you where there are no boundaries between perceived reality and the great beyond. Your spirit is free, and along the path, you find the eternity of the present, the liberation of the past, and with it, the release of suffering. Suffering becomes inappropriate and nonexistent.

Yoga is the action and the strength of our journey.

Yoga has the power to use the present and transform it to a better moment.

In the deep state of human ignorance, we all need to use a little yoga to place ourselves on the path of the true self.

Yoga helps us to live in the present.

The only existing moment we all have is the present. The present is the moment we all share, we all experience. Only in this present exists everything you want, you look, and you deserve. It is only in the now where life is uplifted and enjoyed.

If you look for happiness, you better find it now, at this moment. Don't wait for future happiness and don't live from past happiness. They are both false.

Happiness is a concept, a mental state available to you each moment right now.

Everything is available for you at this moment, right now.

If you are not here, you miss it.

It is as simple and easy as this.

They say we are the creators of our present. Yes, indeed. When things don't go our way, when life seems to give a splash back, we should check whether our minds are in the present or in worries about the future. When your mind is in the present, there is no need for any stress or anxiety because the present is perfection. Life is perfect if you know how to live it. There is no problem at all. Problems in human beings exist in the mind, nowhere else. In the present exists all that there is. In the present exist beauty, unity, perfection, love, harmony, God, the stars, peace, abundance, joy, and all good things you can imagine.

We came to life to enjoy the moment and to be happy, and sometimes we really look for all that is contrary. With just our eyes open, and remembering our goals, we can return to love.

Marta Berry

2016

References and Sources

- *The Yoga Sutras of Patanjali* by B. K. S. Iyengar
- *The Light on Yoga* by B. K. S. Iyengar
- Bhagavad Gita
- *Yoga* by Manuel Morata
- *The New Book of Yoga* by Sivananda
- *Flower Bach* by Edward Bach
- *You Can Do It* by Louise Hay
- *The Detox Solution* by Patricia Fitzgerald
- *Skinny Bitch* by Rory Freedman and Kim Barnoun
- *Anatomy of Movement* by Blandine Calais–Germain

Glossary of Asana

Atma: Supreme Spirit
Ashtanga: The eight limbs of yoga
Avastha: Condition of the mind
Alasya: Laziness
Ananta: The Infinite
Bandha: Engage, seal
Bhakti: Devotion
Bija: Seed
Brahma: The Supreme Power
Buddhi: Intellect, reason
Chandra: Moon
Danava: Demon
Dhenu: Cow
Guru: Spiritual teacher
Himalaya: Mountains in northern India
Japa: Chant or prayer
Jiva: Individual soul
Jivanaa: Life
Kama: Desire
Karuna: Compassion
Kaya: Body
Klesa: Pain, anxiety
Loma: Hair
Man: To think
Moha: Cheating trick
Mudra: Seal, posture
Mukti: Let go, liberate
Prana: Life, energy, vitality
Parvata: Mountain
Prajna: Intelligence, wisdom
Purnata: Perfection

Raja: King
Sadhana: Practice, search
Sadhaka: Aspirant, student
Samsaya: Doubt
Samskara: Impression of the past
Sita: Cold
Surya: Sun
Swami: Master
Tantra: Liberation of mind and body
Vacha: Language
Yukta: One who reaches the union with spirit
Adho: Down
Anga: Limb
Angusta: Big toe
Ardha: Half
Baka: Crane
Bheka: Frog
Bujangha: Serpent
Chandra: Moon
Chatu: Four
Danda: Stick
Dhanu: Bow
EKA: One
Garuda: Eagle
Go: Cow
Hala: Plough
Hanuma: King of monkeys
Hasta: Hand
Janu: Knee
Jathara: Stomach
Kapota: PigeonKARNA—Ear
Kona: Angle
Krouncha: Heron
Kurma: Turtle

Mala: Garland
Matsya: Fish
Marichya: Wise—Sage
Mula: Root
Mudra: To seal
Mukha: Face
Nava: Boat
Nata: Dancer
Pada: Foot
Padma: Lotus
Parivrtta: Revolved
Parigha: Bar
Parisva: Spin
Parsva: Side
Parvata: Mountain
Paschimo: West
Parivrtta: Turn
Pida: Pain
Pincha: Chin
Purvo: East
Raja: King
Salaba: Locust
Sarva: Complete
Setu: Bridge
Sida: Saint
Sirsa: Head
Supta: Lying down
Svana: Dog
Savasa: Corpse
Tada: Mountain
Triko: Three
Tola: Scale
Urdvha: Upward
Ustra: Camel

Utka: Chair
Utta: Intense
Vira: Hero
Vrk: Tree
Vasistha: Wise, Sage

Chapter 1

Methodology of Teaching Yoga

Teaching yoga is a wonderful and privileged profession.

Any person with faith, effort, and altruism can become a yoga instructor. Teaching yoga is about the desire to actively bring a few grains of sand to help stimulate the transformation of someone. It's about helping students reconnect with the divine or with that innate infinity that exists inside each of us.

Namaste, the Indian salutation, means "we all are one and take part in the same big universe together." Spiritually there are no boundaries between human beings. Being a yoga teacher goes beyond just being an instructor in a gymnasium. Becoming a good teacher of yoga requires knowledge of the fundamental aspects of yoga, philosophy, anatomy, and methodology.

The science of yoga focuses on the alignment of asana, biomechanics, and an understanding of movement. Teaching yoga involves modifications and variations of the asana to accommodate the body type and level of the student's conditioning, the respiration, the sequences of classes, as well as the basic organization of classes.

We all have a wonderful teacher inside us. We all have a past and history. We all have karma to clean. The only thing we must do is awaken the sense of desire through inspiration, admiration of beauty, and the innate need to grow spiritually. We must become a reflection for others—not only with words but also with vibrations of love, light, and truth.

We will learn that the easiest way to find ourselves is to get lost in the service of others.

Capture the Energy Level of the Student

An alert mind includes a clear and communicative voice. A teacher is creative and innovative, maintains a fresh and vibrant body, is charismatic, is positive, has a good sense of humor, and is inspiring.

Technique

When you become a yoga instructor, you become a guide to adventures in strength and energy. You need to lend a sense of security to help your students get to a magical place. The yoga teacher wants to use all his or her experiences and technical knowledge to guide the group in a positive manner toward a happy destiny. The success of this journey depends on your ability to connect energetically with the mind, body, and heart of the student. Each student is unique. The challenge for the teacher is simply that the same techniques will not work for everyone.

It is important to be alert, creative, and improvisational. You need to find new ways to motivate, inspire, and educate. Each individual has a certain level at which you can reach him or her to turn the practice into a success. There exists a relationship between the depth of the teachings, the number of students, the feeling in the room, and the level of the teacher's maturity and authority that can be maximized. Your students will sense these levels. They must be able to trust the teacher. When the teacher has experience and knows how to execute the lessons, the teacher can be the most effective. A teacher with experience knows how to cultivate a student's abilities and connect with the largest number of students.

Technical knowledge makes life easier. It also helps you get things done faster and more securely. Technical knowledge comes from training and experience; however, that isn't enough. The teacher must also cultivate his or her own creativity to come up with techniques so he or she can make a connection and develop students. Through this connection, the teacher can transport the student to a magical place where the heart extends with a natural form and where everyone is enriched. The service of teaching yoga truly is a divine privilege. Every student is a gift.

Be in Service

"A pioneer in the relationship of body, mind, and spirit" is a valid description of those who practice yoga in the twenty-first century. Science now tells us that what happens in one part of the body clearly affects all other parts; the corporeal systems are interrelated, and each influences the others.

Even when beginning from the deepest parts of human ignorance, we must learn that the work we do in life is part of the divine will. We should each strive to elevate the deep thoughts of consciousness and offer every one of our daily works to God.

Being a yoga teacher is an act of thankfulness for life and the opportunity we have to work for the prosperity of mankind.

Communication

Our basic communication abilities directly influence all aspects of life; therefore, communication has a direct impact on the process of student learning.

Communication consists of two parts: the transmission of a message and the receipt of the response. Communication may be verbal or nonverbal. Nonverbal communication is transmitted through body language, facial expressions, movements, gestures, and posture. Verbal communication is made through the use of voice, the articulation of words, and terms of expression. Always use plain language so students can understand what you are saying. The secret of successful communication is to ensure that the person you are speaking with understands what is being said.

The way you communicate will influence students' performance. Use descriptive words such as *elongate, activate, open, flow, begin to, sink into, find, stay open, maintain, hold, gaze, lengthen, keep, drawn, remain centered, relax, maneuver, initiate, challenge, find opposition,* and so forth.

Contact

Contact is an indispensable tool for communication. Physical contact lingers in the unconscious physical memory for thirty seconds beyond the moment of touch. Your skin is the largest and most sensitive organ of your body. Receptors in the skin transmit information to the brain via the nervous system. In teaching, we apply contact to muscles and articulating zones, shoulders, and hips. Each student has his or her own way of learning. Be aware of this and give your attention to your students; show them when they are doing the wrong thing and don't be afraid to correct errors.

However, at the same time, you want to promote independence in your students. Let them move! When it comes to asana, teach their bodies, not their minds. Use your sense of humor and transport your students into the present.

Look them in the eyes. Eye contact communicates volumes.

Voice

In yoga instruction, the voice is a key element of communication. Your voice reflects the attitude of your heart. The tone of your voice originates in the heart, not the mind.

Remember—the size of your class should determine the volume of your voice. Volume isn't power. What you have to say and how you choose to say it are the driving factors in your student experience.

The voice must come from the diaphragm, as in singing. If we use vocal cords incorrectly, we can injure ourselves. Relax the vocal cords; learn to speak from the diaphragm. Open your chest and use intonation to produce melody for your sound.

Speak in an adult tone. Unless you are actually teaching children, don't talk to your students as if they were children. Avoid singing. Be enthusiastic, inspiring, amiable, and communicative. Modulate your voice to promote alertness in your class. Synchronize your instruction with the asana you are teaching. Don't forget to breathe between sentences.

When teaching lower-energy classes, the voice must convey a more relaxed state. Try to end your statements using the same energy with which you began them. Speak clearly to create impact with what you say. Keep the class moving but don't forget to use pauses thoughtfully to allow students to truly absorb detailed instructions. When leading a seminar, create pauses so you can rest while demonstrating or explaining. Say something if you see a student making a mistake but be compassionate.

Adjustment

The main reason for adjusting and aligning your students is to help them express the intentions of their spirits and hearts in the best possible manner. This is the end goal and the most profound result of their practices.

A posture is never "good" or "bad." It is instead either in or out of correct alignment. We must always try to find a way to recognize something good in each pose and in each student. We try to find the most basic and obvious misalignments visible in the students' poses as we observe our classes.

The student is the owner of his or her own movements. Each person has his or her own state of physical ability, mental condition, and spiritual level. This is reflected in the learning curve. As professionals, we must respect everyone and fully recognize that each body is a materialization of the divine force. Make no judgments; we are here to help students find the new spaces in their bodies. We are there to help them feel better and become rejuvenated.

Adjustments can be made at all levels, but we should practice restraint when applying adjustments to experienced students of yoga. Beginners appreciate the touch of adjustment, but some experienced students have notions of personal alignment that should be respected.

Making Adjustments

First, it's important to always attempt a verbal correction before attempting physical contact. If you don't know the student, you should always ask for his or her permission before you adjust or touch the body. Once you know the student, adjustments can be made more freely. Ask your student for input on consent; this can change from class to class and from minute to minute.

It isn't necessary to be strict in conducting poses. Moving out and back into asana may help in achieving alignment. Normally you would apply adjustment at articulating areas (joints) such as the hips and shoulders. Also, you may touch the most prominent muscle area in use in the asana (quadriceps, triceps). It is a good idea to demonstrate the breathing that accompanies the asana and the adjustment. Try to show the correct place on the cycle of inhalation and exhalation where the adjustment can be made.

The benefits of yoga come with time and perseverance. Students must feel comfortable and be assured they are progressing in their practice of yoga. Students should never be made to feel they aren't flexible enough, that there is some missing talent required to succeed, that they are wasting their time, or that they have started too late in life.

The two areas of the body that are the most problematic in body alignment are the rib cage and the pelvic area. That is to say that most aches and pains in the musculature tend to occur in these regions. You will serve your clients well if you can help them to develop and maintain the muscles in these two vulnerable areas. Because they are reliant on proper muscular support to function optimally, these areas have considerable influence on posture. They need to be protected and strengthened when in proper alignment.

Alignment

The shoulders and hips support the trunk. The best possible alignment of these areas facilitates the best possible alignments in the asana and the advancement in the abilities of the student. The first asana for proper alignment, the principal aligned position, is the "mountain" pose, Samasthiti or Tadasana. Find this pose in every asana. The principal spinal alignment of this pose reoccurs in all the asana so we are searching for a return to this alignment in moving in and out of all the other asana. We are "pulling the body" into or through Tadasana.

In seated, twisting, and inverted positions, we try to arrive at a partial alignment of Tadasana as can be readily understood through our own practice.

When an asana is repeated, "muscle memory" allows the asana to be more easily reached. When the articulations of the body are in the right alignment, the muscles attached to them naturally establish themselves in the right place and bring success to your work.

To understand alignment, we need to understand the type of the body the pupil has and which form of the asana is performed. Proper alignment comes from the inside of the body and is related to internal energy, the prana, and the mind of the student. If the alignment is only superficial, it will show in a lack of integration of the position.

A dynamic symmetry is the base that connects the interior with the surface of the body.

If the alignment is composed and defined in each aspect, it forms what is called "a blueprint" (the architect's ideal design), and thus, the body learns how to move following the "design" of its own blueprint. It is important to establish the right blueprint to prevent bad habits or lead to injuries.

This blueprint has its very fine energy; it varies between people and during one's lifetime. As we age, the blueprint changes, and it changes as we practice as well. It changes with conscious effort, seeking transformation through exercise and nutrition. In the blueprint of the body, we can also recognize genetics, rhythms, past habits of exercise and rest, and other aspects of life.

When the human body is aligned with its optimal blueprint, the connective tissue (tendons and ligaments where emotional and thick toxins are stored) becomes stronger, more resistant, and flexible; and the internal circulation rises. The human body has an innate intelligence that looks for harmony and health. Normally the body isn't strong enough to align by itself, it needs training through exercise.

Basic points and zones of alignment are the following:

- Base of the pelvis—gluteus
- Abdominal muscles
- Base of the heart
- Shoulder blades to rib cage
- Heels to sitting bones
- Drishti: the focal point where you look
- Kneecaps; lift them up to align quads and hamstrings.
- The alignment of one part of the body has an effect on the others. All body parts are related, and alignment is the foundation of success in movement.
- Big toe: push the bone of the big toe down to awaken and engage the internal activity of the leg.
- Feel every pose from a grounding sensation in opposition.
- Rotation of the hips: internal (heel to heel) or external (heel to arch)

Some Other Tips

A class must hold a student's attention. Run a harmonious class; don't be boring. Don't let your students collapse from fatigue; pace the class so that all stay together. Go to Balasana (child's pose) whenever needed. End each class with a relaxation period and meditation.

Walk: circulate about the class while giving instructions. Watch your students and take the time to observe them. Make sure to assist the students with problems in achieving a pose. Try to connect alignment with breathing. Keep your heart open and smile.

As a teacher, when you demonstrate, make sure everybody can see you.

The process of learning takes three different aspects or phases. These are often called parts of the learning curve:

1. Cognitive to beginner (doesn't know much): complement the students' efforts.
2. Associative to intermediate (knows a little more): start the challenge and recognize improvements.
3. Automat (knows what to do): help to keep mastering the asana and breathing.

Distractions and Obstacles

Yoga, like any other spiritual pursuit, is full of pitfalls and impediments. It is a good idea to look at these so you will know how to overcome them. Above all, we must learn to listen to the voice within and recognize what obstacles are facing us.

1. Vyadhi (bad health). For a yogi, the body is the principal instrument. If the vehicle is broken down, it's impossible for the traveler to continue his or her journey. If the body isn't functioning properly, little active progress can be made. Health is very important because the mind functions in concert with the nervous system. When the body isn't working well, the practice of yoga is interrupted.
2. Styana (mental predisposition). Are you ready to work? When the mental faculties are rusty, progress is difficult. It's important to stay fluid. Don't sit like water in a drain. Keep mentally active.
3. Samsaya (mental paralysis, doubt, and indecision): ignorance and lack of faith, self-destructive tendencies. Joy and happiness cannot be found in these states of mind. You need faith in yourself and in your guru. Trust in the supreme energy to be found in your own interior. Faith strengthens the heart and destroys evil.
4. Pramada (indifference to others); to be totally immersed in your own self-importance, lacking in humility and the belief that you know it all. These characteristics lead to a never-ending, empty pursuit of satisfying base passions and egotistical dreams.

5. Alasaya (laziness): to triumph over laziness, one must apply will and enthusiasm, and find hope. The attitude of the student must be one of a person in love, full of hope and free of hate and pain. Faith and an enthusiasm for life conquer laziness.
6. Avirati (liberation from the pleasures that trap your mind): emancipate yourself from empty desires.
7. Bhranti-darsana (wrongful thought): wrongful thoughts empower wrongful wisdom.
8. Alabdha-bhumikatva (inability to concentrate): This named obstacle promotes an inability to find reality. If you can't see with clarity, you go around crashing into things and continue a train of thought that isn't real.
9. Anavasthitatva (instability to maintain what you have). Unhealthy pride in your own abilities leads to abandonment.
10. Find the way to be happy and overcome these obstacles—seek benevolence, unity, compassion, and charity.

Benefits

The purpose of yoga, the resulting state of the practice of yoga and its power, is the complete liberation from contact with the world of suffering, pain, and affliction. Nothing exists higher than this power. It is like a sparkling, perfectly cut diamond that offers the brilliant light of all colors. Yoga possesses diverse facets that reflect the energy of the life-force into its distinct and beautiful forms to create inner peace and happiness.

The privilege of the human being is work, not its fruits. To work with the desire to achieve the divine—to come closer to God, as is sometimes said—and to abandon all desire and egoism, yoga is the union between force and desire.

The practice of yoga reinforces the musculature and nervous system. It brings serenity and permits the student to develop a new perspective of wisdom, a vision less terrestrial and more cosmic. It awakens joy and brings light into the daily life, beaming this light from the interior, from the life-force of the student, out to the greater world.

Yoga vitalizes the circulatory, respiratory, skeletal-muscular, endocrine, dermal, nervous, and lymphatic systems.

Yoga fortifies all the muscles of the body and releases stiffness in the neck, shoulders, and extremities. It brings agility and lightness. It rejuvenates, elongates the spine, and returns energy and mobility to the body. It improves digestion and alleviates gastric disorders. It expands the chest while eliminating anxiety and depression.

Yoga cures insomnia, quells unnecessary desires, activates the glands, and aids and improves the functioning of the organs. After a good session of yoga, the body is newly awakened. With practice, little by little, a new perspective is born, and the student advances a little further into the world of personal discovery and finds the desire, the need, to know more, to want to improve and activate a little more of the innate sense of the mystical we all possess.

Suggestions and Advice for the Study of Yoga

To practice yoga is to feed the spirit; yoga requires strength (mental and physical). The principals of Yamas and Niyamas form the basic elements of the study of yoga.

The aspiring yogi must apply himself or herself to reinforce self-discipline, faith, tenacity, and perseverance for the practice.

On a practical level, one may achieve asana most easily after bathing and emptying one's intestines. Asana are best practiced on an empty stomach. Hydrating—drinking tea, water, and juices—before practice is recommended.

The best time of the day to practice asana is in the first hours of the morning or in the afternoon at and following sunset. A morning session prepares your day, giving you power in your daily work. An afternoon session aids in dissipating the daily stress and leaves the body relaxed and supple for a refreshing sleep.

During practice, relax and release all tension in the muscles of the face, the temples and jaw, ears, and eyes. Relax your breathing.

Practice is made with eyes open; in this way the student is able to see for focusing, for balancing, and for helping to achieve the poses—to see

11

errors while learning. Once the asana has been mastered, the eyes may be closed for a deeper feeling of the stretching, elongating, and opening of the muscles and organs.

Movement cures, heals, and purifies—movement occurs throughout the body. During practice the entire body is active; the mind is passive yet awake. Respiration is best when affected through the nose.

Savasana is the proper way to conclude a session of yoga. It dissipates tension and fatigue after a strenuous, energetic practice.

A proper yoga session is well proportioned in its asana and is light and joyful. The session permits the student to establish a unity between body, mind, and spirit. Once the asana are learned and fully achieved, they will become familiar with practice and become easy for the body, free of force and problems.

Metaphorically, the body will adopt diverse shapes—from the shape of the most insignificant insect to that of the greatest of beasts to that of the wisest of yoga masters. The yogis know that all things exist in their own phase of a natural process of life and that we all breathe in the same air, the prana, of the Universal Spirit. In this way we develop our interior focus and learn to feel the presence of God in our own bodies as we travel through each asana.

With this interior awakening, we comprehend true power, and this creates within us the need to become servants of the divine—of this power—offering all we have and achieve.

Through this intricate coordination of forces concentrated in our bodies, together with the feelings of the mind and reasoning, the human being obtains the grand prize—inner peace and communion of his or her spirit with God.

Injuries

In the path of yoga, injury must be considered a possibility. The instructor must be aware that injuries visit the body for many different reasons. Injuries can result from softening actions or performance, from students not learning how to listen carefully to the body's needs, from the need to burn impurities from life, from erasing karma, or from other aspects of a student's life.

The yogi/yogini should note, however, that as injuries arrive, they can sometimes arrive for the good. Once the injury disappears, the area may become stronger, more flexible, and pain free. It's important to have a sense of gratitude for the pain instead of a sense of complaining and not accepting it.

Take good care; limit the intake of sugar, refined flours, and dead animals as much as packaged food. Find alternative remedies, such as massage and radio-wave therapy. Apply arnica creams in affected areas and have faith that nothing last forever.

Bandhas

The bandhas are specific points in the body related directly to muscles, through which the prana is transmitted from the centers of the body, the chakras. As energy transmission point zones, they are also areas where adjustments are made in executing asana to achieve alignment for best prana flow.

Mula Bandha

This is the important lowest bandha in the very root of the body, the genital and anal areas and the pelvic "floor." This bandha is like a doorway that lets the prana in and also holds it in the body from escaping.

Uddiyana Bandha

The second bandha, located just below the area of the navel, is the energetic zone of the transverse abdominal muscles and key internal organs. Uddiyana bandha delivers prana to the diaphragm and in all directions in the body, feeding prana to the internal organs up to the stomach and the lower parts of the lungs. The prana is simply related not only to the muscles but also to the function of cleaning and clarifying the internal organs.

Jalandhara Bandha

The zone of this vital bandha is from the chin to the sternum, and it serves the lungs and heart; therefore it is important for blood flow. It also feeds prana to the glands in the throat and imparts prana via the major flow of blood to the head and brain.

Maha Bandha—The Great Center

(The three bandhas are activated at the same time)

During the activity of pranayama, the bandhas help to activate the energy and seal it into the body. It is in this state that the mysterious and powerful current is generated that penetrates Sushumna, allowing kundalini to rise.

Mula bandha circulates the energy in the lower regions, while uddiyana bandha carries it upward to where jalandhara bandha seals it in; the vessel of the body is full. This awakens kundalini–Shakti, and the enlightenment begins in the lower chakras and proceeds upward.

The prana is stored in Manipura Chakra (solar plexus)

Class Sequence

Vinyasa yoga is a style where someone creates his or her sequences.

At first when you begin teaching classes, it is important to make an outline or guide of the asana you will be teaching. Outlines will include instructions on how to perform the asana and its benefits as well as a list of parts of the body affected and so forth. Consider this a normal step in class preparation.

Each yoga class should have a progression, which moves all muscles of the body (Sun Salutation). After focus the practice as you want to create them on a specific set of positions (standing poses, balanced poses, forward folds, back bends, and so forth), including all type of categories and advancing through asana in a progressive manner—easy to more energetic, complicated, and difficult—and finish with a well-deserved Savasana

It is strongly recommended that you construct your first classes in sequences that won't lead to distractions and ensure that a class will stay on track and not take a turn toward positions you don't want your students to go into. Later, with more experience and confidence, your classes can tend to flow themselves with a more spontaneous progression of asana—meaning a less structured preparation of classes.

A good yoga instructor develops the intuitive skill to recognize and discover the level of the class and lead through the asana that is most beneficial for them, using the yogi's own teaching style. The only way to maintain your ability to teach others is with your own regular practice.

Vinyasa Format

Here is the typical sequence for a yoga class:

Opening

- Find a seated position.
- Center the body and breath.
- Give class opening instruction—words to create intention, meditation (these may include a mantra, song, and so forth) Aum.
- Do session of pranayama (optional).

Warm-Up

Warm-up typically includes some preliminary stretching of neck, shoulders, arms, back, lateral core muscles, legs, and so forth. This is usually done in a more-or-less controlled form led by the instructor and may include controlled breathing. Warm-up teaches the teacher the condition of the student.

- Tadasana—recenter the body, talk about bandhas, dedicate the practice, and breathe in the form Ujjayi pranayama.

Sun Salutation A, B (always Ashtanga style)

- Sun Salutation circulates energy through the entire body.

Asana—practice of poses as the instructor sequences them

- Standing positions
- Balance positions
- Back bends
- Forward folds to sitting positions
- Hip openers to shoulder openers
- Twists
- Arm balancing
- Abdominal work
- Inverted positions

Conclusion of Class

- General stretching
- Meditation
- Savasana
- Songs or repeated mantras
- Lesson, teaching, affirmation, and so forth Aum.
- Final remarks—words of gratitude, light, strength, value, and hope
- Namaste

Description—A Classic Yoga Session

A classic session of yoga opens the heart and mind. It may begin in any one of a number of ways. There are yoga teachers who, after warm-up and opening remarks, like to begin with arm stretches and hip openers. Others begin directly with the Sun Salutation and from there carry on with a standing asana. There is no absolute rule that must be followed in sequencing a class; however, as mentioned above, classes should include all types or categories of asana—to use and awaken energy in all parts of the body. As the yoga instructor, you decide how to make your class flow and seek the asana you feel are most appropriate and beneficial for your students.

The practice of yoga isn't easy; you mold your body and mind, and as an instructor, you facilitate this in your students. Students of yoga (yogis) may discover yoga later in life. Beginning after the age of forty isn't uncommon and is, in fact, ideal for maintaining health, promoting longevity, preventing ailments, and embarking on a holistic lifestyle.

Someone has said, "Curiosity erases the footprints of fear." Yoga doesn't create restrictions; yoga unlocks curiosity. Yoga isn't about physical flexibility; it's about knowledge, about discovering the true self that resides within each of us. Yoga is a mystical pursuit. The goal of yoga is to live in love, to discover the God force in our very interior. To find this light, we must pass through the shadows. God is everywhere and in all things; we must learn to be present, to be here in the moment. And in this way we find the true mysticism, the mystic moment in which we live.

One must learn that from within the shadows of life lies a great opportunity. Yoga is an invitation to understand change, love, and fear. Yoga is about these things; it is about something mystical inside you. Yoga is what helps you see what can and cannot be seen.

Love is always more powerful than fear. With yoga, we learn to establish the connection between our bodies, minds, and spirits. We learn that everything at one level has an effect on everything at each of the other levels. It follows, then, that what we eat and drink is as important as the thoughts that come into our minds, the words that come out of our mouths, and the actions we take through our daily lives.

The practice of yoga is a personal revelation in which deep fears, insecurities, and instability are brought to the surface, dealt with, and cast off. Yoga is a place where we see where we can go by simply maintaining our breath and being in the present.

The perfection of the asana comes when it is natural and requires no force at all.

Experience will bring harmony in your classes. Begin with structure; once you have established your experience, you may begin to depart from the need for a prepared, structured format. You will have learned to recognize what your classes need in each moment.

Sharing and Unity

Yoga isn't an activity you do for yourself alone; the word *yoga* means "unity," and this sense of unity should be reflected into the community. In other words, you share your practice. In this way, when people practice yoga, they must understand that their practice is a blessing and for the benefit of their family, friends, and community in general. Yoga is founded in the philosophy that "we are all one." Naturally, the yoga practitioner is strengthening and feeding his or her body during the class, but the benefit of the energy generated is for the good of all humankind.

Pranayama

Pranayama is the fourth limb of yoga and is composed of breathing-technique exercise designed to calm the fluctuations of the mind. The best way to calm the mind is through the perfection of the practice of pranayama. Let's break the work down into its parts.

Prana—life, energy, light, and power
Yama—control

Pranayama means control over the life-force. *Prana* is the energy used by the spirit. This force animates the matter of all things in this material world.

Pranayama consists principally of three phases:

Inspiration—Puraka
Retention—Kumbhaka
Exhalation—Rechaka

We develop intelligence in the body through asana. After we have reached the body, we reach the mind with the deep practice of pranayama. This permits the body to be agile, the mind alert, and the spirit awake.

In the practice of pranayama, we use the lungs as tools for work. For this reason it is necessary that the respiratory system be clean, that the lungs have proper care, and that we learn how to use them correctly.

The best time for practicing pranayama is in the early morning.

A strict and devoted yogi will take at least fifteen minutes to practice pranayama in the early morning. Pranayama should be practiced in a clean, airy place, with clean air free of dust and insects, and in maximum silence if possible.

The postures for this practice are Siddhasana, Virasana, Padmasana, and Baddha Konasana. Any other sitting pose may be used as long as the spine is maintained in alignment.

The practice of pranayama is made without force; the muscles of the face, eyes, and ears are totally relaxed. The neck, shoulders, arms, legs and feet—the entire body is relaxed; the tongue is passive and comfortable inside the mouth.

During any pranayama session, the chin should be above the sternum and clavicle, maintaining jalandhara bandha active. The eyes should be closed. The yogi clears his or her mind of worries and focuses on feeling the life-force without any doubt.

The continued practice of pranayama transforms the mental perspective of the practitioner and his or her attachments to the stresses associated with things of the world, including his or her own habits and addictions.

Suggestions and advice for the practice of pranayama

- Practice regularly.
- Clean the nostrils.
- Relax facial muscles.
- Don't attempt to exceed the capacity of your lungs.
- Don't talk, eat, or drink during the practice.
- Practice with concentration.
- Sing a song or chant a mantra prior to beginning.
- Bless your spiritual master before beginning.
- Practice with patience and calm serenity.
- Maintain the bandhas engages.

Prana isn't limited to air (it isn't physically air); it is life-giving energy. It is found in food, water, sunlight, starlight, and so forth. The highest form of prana is thought, the activity that comes out of consciousness. Prana has the function and capacity to destroy infirmity in the body. When we practice pranayama, we learn the ability to store the life-force energy of Manipura Chakra (solar plexus). With frequent and sustained practice, pranayama incrementally improves your power of control, concentration, and moral character; and it advances your spiritual evolution.

The Path to Establish Pranayama

- Inhale for the count of five, retain for the count of five, exhale for the count of five, and retain for the count of five.
- Repeat this cycle a few times until the body relaxes.

The Three Yogi Respirations

- Breathe in and seal the breath at the bottom of the belly.
- Breathe in and seal the breath at the bottom of the stomach.
- Breathe in and seal the breath at the bottom of the lungs.

Anuloma Viloma (ten rounds)

For Anuloma Viloma pranayama, use the right hand. Bend the first two fingers and place the ring finger on the left nostril and the thumb in the right nostril.

Pinch the right nostril and exhale through the left nostril. Breathe in through the left nostril, pinch both nostrils, and hold the air inside the lungs. Open the right nostril and breathe out, then breathe in through the right nostril. Pinch both nostrils and hold the air; open the left nostril and breathe out. This is one round.

This pranayama is a preparation for the other deeper pranayama techniques and is the technique that provides a deep purification of the nadis.

The timing varies depending on the level of the practitioner. Normally start with a count of inhalation for two, retention for six, and exhalation for four.

When we reach a greater capacity in the lungs, we may use a count of inhalation for four, retention for eight, and exhalation for six.

In this pranayama exercise, the blood receives a better supply of oxygen in both lobes of the mind for a refreshing feeling, nerves are calmed and purified, and the mind becomes tranquil and lucid.

Remember the bandhas.

Kapalbhati (three rounds): Abdominal Respiration of Fire

We get the word *kapalbhati* through the following:

Kapal, "the mind"
Bhati, "to shine"

This pranayama is also called the "breath of fire." It is a very powerful technique for cleaning the organic system of the body.

Take a deep breath, filling the lungs with air. Allow the abdomen to initiate the breathing cycle. Inhale and exhale in a rhythmic manner as the abdomen pumps in and out.

After repeating about fifty force exhalations, let the rest of the air flow out through the nose. Inhale deeply and stay in Kumbhaka state for fifteen seconds. Afterward, exhale completely through the nose and breathe normally.

Kapalbhati invigorates the abdominal region (muscles and organs) such as the pancreas and liver; it clears the nasal passages and refreshes the eyes.

Remember the bandhas.

Ujjayi Pranayama

We get the word *Ujjayi* through the following:

U, "to expand"
Jai, "victory"

In a conscious manner, we learn to be aware of our breathing by listening to and controlling its flow. Ujjayi breathing is a unique technique in which we create the sound of the ocean inside of us, and with this technique, we practice asana. This is done by breathing in deeply through the nose and exhaling through the nose, allowing the air to travel to the back of the throat, across the vocal cords, and to the deepest part of the larynx. Note the sound of the wave of air (like the ocean) as it passes out between the palette and tongue.

This sound is a reflection of our lives, an imprint, the fact of our existence made manifested by our respiration. If we concentrate on this sound, we can find significance in our existence, in our practice. This particular pranayama creates heat in the body and dissolves toxins in the circulatory system.

Ujjayi pranayama aerates the lungs, expels mucus, generates endurance in the body, calms the nerves, and is a tonic for the entire organism. Feel the breath toward mula bandha in and out, conquering the spine's length.

Sitali Pranayama (ten rounds)

In Sitali pranayama, the mouth is open, and the tongue is shaped as a tube, the sides touching the teeth and extended out over the lips.

- Inhale through the open mouth and across the tongue, provoking a sound of "sesee," until the lungs are completely filled. When the lungs are full, retract your tongue and close your mouth. Lower your head, practice jalandhara bandha, and hold the breath for ten seconds—Kumbhaka. Then breathe out through the nose.
- Repeat the cycle ten to twenty times. At the end, lay down to rest in Savasana. This pranayama refreshes the body and cools it down. It is especially good for the eyes and ears, and it also activates the liver and improves the digestive system.

Sitkari Pranayama (ten rounds)

This pranayama is similar to Sitali. It has the same benefits but uses a different position of the tongue.

- Roll the tongue up inside the mouth so the tip barely touches the palette.
- Breathe in through the mouth, provoking the sound "sssss." Close the mouth, holding the air inside; perform jalandhara bandha and hold the breath for ten seconds. Then exhale slowly through the nose.
- Repeat the cycle ten to twenty times. At the end, gently assume Savasana.

The Lion Breath (five rounds)

Deeply inhale through the nose and exhale. Open the mouth and stick the tongue out, rolling the eyes upward. The practice of the Lion Breath clears and cleanses the throat.

History, Paths and Styles of Yoga

The word *yoga* in Sanskrit means "union." Yoga is most simply and commonly defined as "the true union of the individual will with the God's will." The concept of God can also be related to a "True Reality," "Highest Power." "Universal Power," "Divine Light" "Creator," and so forth. In yoga, the human being comprises body, mind, and spirit; and the aim or result of practice is a more perfect union of these three entities as a natural process in achieving union with God.

In the practice of yoga, each yogi has his or her own realization of where he or she is on the path to this union—to this enlightenment—based on his or her practice, the effort put forward, and his or her sense of his or her own interior peace and happiness.

Your privilege is work, not its fruits.

Yoga History

The origins of Yoga are lost in the annals of remotest time. Yoga is considered a divine science of life revealed to enlighten wise men through meditation. Archeologists have found the oldest rock art representing figures in yoga positions in the stones of the Indus Valley, dating to approximately 3,000 BC.

The earliest mention of yoga is found in the Vedas, the vast collection of sacred writings of India, dating back as early as 2,500 BC. The pillars of yoga teachings are found in the Upanishads, which form the ultimate parts of the Vedas.

In the Vedas we encounter the concept of Brahman, which represents the absolute, the complete universe.

In the sixth century, 600 BC, two epic poems appear: Pranayama and Mahabharata. The Mahabharata contains the Bhagavad Gita, perhaps the best-known piece of Indian literature in Yoga. In the Bhagavad Gita, Brahman (in the form of Krishna) instructs the warrior Arjuna about yoga, and specifically he describes the way to reach liberation and complete the tasks of life. We also have the teachings of the yoga sutras of Patanjali, texts that date from 300 BC.

Yoga is the union of Shiva and Brahman (the divine absolute consciousness) with Jiva (the individual being).

Four Paths of Yoga: Karma, Bhakti, Jnana, and Raja

Karma Yoga (The Yoga of Action, Yoga Is Life)

Exhibiting dedication to others and selfless action, karma-yoga is a daily labor; beyond the teachings or techniques of yoga, we learn the correct approach to yoga, how to think about yoga. In karma-yoga we learn that in this life all take part of yoga.

It isn't what you have or where you are on the path that is important; what matters is your approach to yoga—to the liberation, the motivation behind the practice. It must be pure.

The true work of life is to be directed toward God, the divine, that which is inside and is the master of the universe. We learn through the circumstances and experiences life brings us. Our work should be directed in gratitude to what gives us life.

The Teachings: To Do One's Best

Do and labor the best you can, in all things in the best way you know how. Don't permit fear or laziness in your laboring. Develop actions (habits and thoughts) that promote good to the maximum and limit the negative to the possible minimum.

The Teachings: Let the Results Go

God, not you, is the one who does things. You are simply an instrument, and in the most profound sense, you cannot know the nature or intentions of God. The true "I" is unchanging; what is changing are the gunas, the three qualities or properties of nature. This truth is realized when the yogi recognizes that the truth is the work—constant work— abandoning the results of the actions. The desire to act or the desire for action creates the individual. This is a profound concept that forms the basis and sows the seeds of karma (the cosmic law of cause and effect). To give up, give away, or simply let stand the results of your actions is the greatest liberation; it means you are working freely. Understand that the results of work are neither inferior nor superior; they are simply the results. Don't be attached to them; instead prepare to go on, to change. Simply stated, in all you do, stay alert to the truth that you are serving God, serving the divine power.

The Golden Rule—do unto others as you would have them do unto you—applies to karma-yoga. Adapt, accommodate; to insult and be argumentative is to wound. *Unity* means unity with all—honor and diversity; we are all part of the same body. Practice humility of heart. These are actions; these are the teachings of yoga of action, karma-yoga.

Follow the discipline of labor. Every task is its master. In karma-yoga, you see things from the perspective that you learn specific things from specific types of work—the work teaches you. Therefore, the yogi should search for concentration, experience, emotional reinforcement, and physical energy. Search out work that suits you, that you will like, and be the best at it. Then work with love and gusto.

Bhakti Yoga: The Yoga of Devotion

Bhakti yoga is the yoga of speech and the heart, sacred song, and lengthy and continuous meditation. Bhakti yoga is discussed further in the philosophy section.

Jnana-Yoga: The Yoga of Wisdom

Jnana-yoga is the yoga of knowledge and wisdom. It is the enlightenment achieved through knowledge and truth, the process of learning, the understanding of the concepts of the highest wisdom, the power of vision and liberation of total understanding. It is the way of personal revelation and comprehension of truth (enlightenment). The masters of jnana-yoga assert that all that is real exists in the consciousness and consider that there is no separation between consciousness and the universe. There is no distinction between consciousness and reality, and true illumination occurs when there is true union, not merely a mental exercise but union of the spirit of the yogi with the Universal Spirit. This is the discovery of Atman (the soul) in its pure spiritual state, separate from mind and body, beyond the realm of thoughts or the physical world. It masters the cultivation of knowledge through philosophers and mediators.

Power of will and inspired reason are the pillars of jnana-yoga, which is practiced by meditation, self-observation, consciousness, study, and reflection.

Raja-Yoga: The Physical Yoga

The Royal Path—our yoga, the physical practice, the combination of asana, pranayama, meditation, development of control of body and mind. He who practices this yoga follows the path of Patanjali.

Explore the mind and the consciousness. The journey travels from the interior to the exterior world, with the goal of understanding the nature of the being and its infinite potential.

Different Styles of Yoga

Different styles make the practice of yoga a truly full experience. As a yogi, it is interesting to be familiar with the different styles of yoga that, with the passage of time, have come out of the root of hatha-yoga.

Hatha

All of yoga is hatha—hatha is the mother. A class or session of hatha-yoga includes pranayama, meditation, and asana. Let's look at the meaning of *hatha*: Ha, "sun"; tha (moon equilibrium between sun and moon).

Sun Salutation—different opening launches

Ashtanga (Pattajabhi Jois)

This is the system of yoga that means the "eight limbs or aspects" of yoga. Ashtanga yoga follows the series of A, B, C, and D, which integrates power and grace. It requires a distinct level of flexibility and humility. Each asana prepares the yogi for the next asana in a progression in a meticulous practice.

Drishti, the practice of having the eyes fixed on focal points during the practice, is used. There are nine drishti; these include the nose, between the brows, the navel, the index fingers, hands, feet, and positions to the right and left sides. Drishti stabilizes and purifies the mind. Ashtanga is a pure and traditional method of yoga that requires daily practice focusing on the posture, the breath, and the drishti.

Vinyasa

Vinyasa is a kind of yoga that embraces different traditions such as Ashtanga, Iyengar, and Vini yoga. It is a style in which one asana flows into the next. During the practice, the motion between the asana is fluid, relaxed yet precise, a form of active meditation. Each breath accompanies a dynamic movement. To correctly practice vinyasa, the student must first learn each asana independently. The synchronization of the breathing with the movement through the asana promotes cardiovascular activity; the effort heats the blood for improved circulation and cleansing of toxins in the body, the articulating portions of the body particularly, as well as the digestive track. The body is refreshed, strong, and supple. Drishti is also practiced in vinyasa yoga.

Bikram (Hot Yoga)

The master Bikram Choudhury created Bikram, also known as "hot yoga." In Bikram the room is heated to 40 degrees Celsius. The muscles become elastic, and flexibility is increased. Also at this hot temperature, the body is induced to sweat and release toxins out of the body. This is a very intense form of yoga and is meant to produce perspiration for cleansing; a full session includes twenty-six asana in a repetition two times through. The first time is for alignment, and the second is to deepen into the stretch. This practice raises issues related to blood pressure, and caution must be used.

Kundalini

In this style, pranayama and sacred songs are performed. In the initial phase of the practice, attention is focused on energy in the base of the spine. Breathing is coordinated with the asana as in vinyasa.

Kundalini is about awakening the inner enlightenment. The exercises are called kriyas (actions, efforts). In the Hindu tradition, kundalini is a spiritual science that, with the help of a guru as a guide, leads to illumination and God's revelations

Iyengar

B. K. S. Iyengar, yoga master, created his own style of yoga in which each asana is performed for a longer period of time. A pose may be held for several minutes with controlled breathing. Accessories such as blocks and straps may be used.

Anusara

Anusara is a practice of hatha-yoga created by modern master John Friend. *Anusara* means "flowing with grace, with nature, from the heart." This yoga is about viewing yoga as an art form. Union is approached through meditation on the eternal beauty and grace of the divine inner light of the heart.

The philosophy of Anusara is about aligning self with the divine power, and through this we achieve union with the Supreme Being. On the physical level in this meditation, we develop fluidity and grace.

Through the power of this grace, we awaken the true fluidity and grace of our true sacred natures.

On the yoga mat, we perform asana while concentrating on the artistic shapes they take, offering the individual light and music of the heart, full of song, beauty, love, and the bond with the world.

Other interesting styles are: Forrest yoga, Integral yoga, Jivamukti yoga, Laughter yoga, Naked yoga, Raja yoga, Rocket yoga, Sivananda yoga, Taoist yoga, Viniyoga, yoga for disorders, and Zen yoga among others.

Final Relaxation: Guided Savasana

The Corpse Pose

Lying on your back, extend your arms long with the hands facing up. Separate the legs mat-width distance apart and turn the feet sideways.

Take a long inhalation through the nose, and as you exhale, sigh out of the mouth.

Feel the under part of the shoulders on the floor and breathe into the space you create across your chest.

Feel yourself open and as symmetrical as possible.

Savasana is also called "pose of surrender," so let the physical body take the quality of surrender from head to toe.

Release areas of tension; maintain a gentle breath so you can rest deeply.

Become fully aware to absorb the benefits of the practice. Settle it down within you and allow the practice to become part of you.

In corpse pose there is nothing left to do. Do nothing and let everything else happen.

Relax the back of the arms, neck, and legs; rest deeply. Feel the hands away from the shoulders and the feet away from the hips.

Soften every part of the body as you become still and as quiet as possible. Feel the floor beneath you and the entire body release. Let it go; remain to your body to let it go. Let go of problems—trauma, drama, complaints, disappointments, even victimization feelings—and just approach the feeling of your inner power and peace. This feeling is here with you, and it is always willing to help you in any desired direction you need.

Soften the breath and rest deeply.

Turn the intention inside, relax deeply, and allow the muscles in the body to relax. With every exhalation go deeper inside; the entire muscles feel soft. The bones are heavy. The more you allow your belly to relax, the more your legs will relax. The better you can relax your muscles, bones, tendons, ligaments, tissues, and so forth, the stronger they will become.

Keep on turning inside more and more; the waves of the breath move you away from the body. Stay with the light. Bathe yourself in the light and suspend yourself in the light—vast, luminous, open, and free.

May all the beings be free of suffering, poverty, ignorance, insecurities, judgments, and fears. May we all discover the high self of our divine infinity.

Let this sensation fill from right to left side, from above on down, shimmering all around. Continue to relax into your own light and bow into the light within you.

Play with the inner relaxations of the skin, legs, shoulders, feet, and top of the head.

And then just recognize one more time the privilege and fortune of being alive today so you can feel the light and, with this enlightenment, feel the gratitude of the moment. Remembering again and again the substance that allows you to live in grace, feel gratitude for who you are, for what you have, and for where you are today.

Gratitude is the basic key to stay in tune with the divine and to find harmony and prosperity. As soon as we lose the vibration of gratitude, disconnection and discontentment arrive. Forgive yourself for not being perfect and forgive others for not understanding you. Develop your devotion; learn how to find reflection of your actions. Without reflection there is no progress. We must understand our mission, appreciate our qualities, and lead ourselves to accomplish whatever we think is possible.

To develop faith with God, it is especially important to maintain acceptance and understand God's will.

Inhale and exhale three times—cleansing breaths through the mouth.

Inhale and stretch arms overhead, feet together; bend knees to the chest, roll side to side, roll to the right, come to a sitting position, keep eyes closed, and sing a blessing.

Namaste—the light within me salutes, respects, and honors the light within you.

Yoga and Pregnancy

- Sun Salutation (modified, hip-width distance)
- Use blocks. Avoid movement of prone position; instead practice Cat-Cow and Adho Mukha Svanasana.
- Yoga is a safe, simple, and natural method of preparing the pregnant woman for motherhood and the baby for childbirth.
- The practice cultivates acceptance, peace, and harmony for the entire family. Yoga is a great way to keep fit during pregnancy, to align your body optimally for healthy carriage and delivery of the baby, to provide breathing and relaxation techniques to use during pregnancy and labor, and to reduce discomfort in the upper and lower back that sometimes accompanies carrying a baby before and after pregnancy. It's best for you to study with a teacher who has training and experience with the ever-changing pregnant body. Ideally it's best to find a prenatal yoga class to help you stay within safe parameters at each stage of your pregnancy. If you are new to yoga and pregnant, ask your doctor or midwife whether a prenatal yoga class would benefit you. However, if you have high blood pressure or other complications in your pregnancy, it's extremely important to check first before starting with the yoga practice.

Basic Asana for Pregnancy

- Sun Salutation A–B—use a chair.

- Cat-Cow—lengthen the legs to the back.
- Trikonasana—use blocks for balance.
- Anjaneyasana—launches—modified with gentle back bend and twist.
- Cobra standing
- Balancing poses (use wall)
- Easy twists—gently stretch arms to sides and up.
- Half Ustrasana and Balasana—only during first and second trimester
- Balasana—spread knees apart. Avoid pressure on the baby; use a bolster for support.
- Paschimottanasana—with legs apart
- Janu Sirsasana—with wide legs
- Baddha Konasana—easy twists with blanket under seat bones
- Upavistha Konasana—use a blanket on the sitting bones for better comfort.
- Sarvangasana—use the wall for support.
- Halasana—use a chair. If the student suffers from heartburn, stay away from performing this pose. Use legs against a wall. This asana has the same benefits as inverted poses.
- Setu Bandhasana—bridge position; use blocks underneath lower back.
- Squats—all movements requiring squatting should be approached carefully.
- Savasana—position body on the left side with knees bent.
- During pregnancy many changes occur in a woman's body and mental state. The growing weight of the baby and the increased amount of blood in the body necessitate more physical training, both to stimulate the blood circulation and counteract fatigue. She also needs to relax, to feel the child in the womb, and to be able to accept her reactions and trust her own sentiments.
- Circulation problems can cause leg pain. It is suggested that a pregnant mom put her legs up to the wall. Folding a blanket and placing it over the bolster, let the head rest on it.

- Massage the souls of the feet to improve circulation, practice plenty of Cat–Cow movements and squats in each session, especially during the second and third trimesters. Encourage walk and rest. After the baby is born, the new mom and baby should start attending postpartum classes.
- If a pregnant lady comes to your class and has never practice yoga, encourage her to find prenatal classes.
- However, if one of your students becomes pregnant, she can probably keep attending your classes, following modifications, and later can be guided to find a prenatal class for her own benefit.
- Remember that pregnancy may include emotional ups and downs that might seem overwhelming at times. Change of moods, depression, managing stress, and anxiety.

Suggestions in Cases of Extra Stress or Anxiety While the Pregnancy Advances

- Cut back on chores—use that time to put your feet up, take a nap, or read a book.
- Take advantage of vacation whenever possible. Spending a day—or even an afternoon—resting at home will help you get through a tough week.
- Try deep-breathing exercises like yoga or stretch muscles.
- Get regular exercise such as swimming or walking.
- Do your best to eat a healthy, well-balanced diet to keep the right energy level.
- Go to bed early. The body is working overtime to nourish your growing baby, and it probably needs more rest and sleep.
- Don't believe everything you hear or read about pregnancies; every woman is different.

Yoga Benefits for Pregnancy

- It improves posture and flexibility.

- It offers extra time to be with the baby.
- It helps to improve self-confidence in the respiration level to prepare for labor.
- It relaxes the mind and helps one to sleep better.
- It helps with uncomfortable pregnancy states as a reduction of swallow ankles and puffy legs.
- It avoids edema, retention of fluids, cramps, and common symptoms of the last trimester.
- It helps with the right position of the baby (it turns the baby around and places the baby's head in its right place).
- It promotes right digestion and good elimination.
- It elevate energy level and helps to maintain active metabolism.
- It helps to reduce nausea and change of mood.

Hints for the Practice

- Drink all the water needed for the practice.
- Don't practice strong twist positions.
- Don't practice with lots of intensity through long periods of time.
- Don't retain the air inside; don't practice Kapalbhati Pranayama, which will produce too much heat for the mother and baby.
- Practice Ujjayi pranayama through the mouth if it is necessary.
- Teach pregnant women how to listen to their bodies and practice with care, with love connecting with the baby, so they can understand that the practice is for both.
- Avoid overstretching.

Partner Yoga

Partner yoga is a fun way to practice yoga with your friends, partner, or children. Almost all the asana can be adapted for a yoga partner. This presentation is an introduction to partner yoga and will help you create playfulness with asana in standing and sitting positions.

Standing Positions

- Tadasana—back to back
- Urdhva Mukha Sirsasana—back to back, with hands touching
- Uttanasana—back to back while grabbing the shins of the partner
- Ardha Uttanasana—back to back or face-to-face, grab arms, forming a bridge with feet together and feet separate.
- Adho Mukha Svanasana—resting the back feet together and feet separately
- Utkatasana—back to back, sitting down and touching hands
- Anjaneyasana—back to back, touching the hands above the head, knees on the floor
- Half Moon—sideways toward inside with legs straight and both arms up or one arm up and the other down
- Virabhadrasana II—back to back, touching hands
- Ardha Chandrasana V—back to back, touching hands
- Parvottanasana—side to side, inside foot together
- Parivrtta Trikonasana—back to back, inside foot together
- Utthita Trikonasana—back to back, different sides
- Utthita Parsvakonasana—back to back, different sides
- Standing up face-to-face—back bend, holding wrists
- Prasarita Padottanasana—back to back, fingers interlaced, head to head and face-to-face (some other modifications)
- Digasana—face-to-face, grabbing the shoulders

Balancing

- Vrksasana—side to side, holding bodies
- Natarajasana—face-to-face, grabbing shoulders
- Utthita Padangusthasana—side to side, holding bodies

Kneeling and Sitting Positions

- Kneeling down, face-to-face, hands touching in Namaste

- Kneeling down, sitting on partner's hips, and leaning back
- Dandasana—back to back, backs touching
- Balasana—head to head
- Paschimottanasana—face-to-face, holding hands or forearms and stretching back and forth, resting on the back with bent knees or straight legs

Hip Openers

- Baddha Konasana—face-to-face, with partner with wide, long legs pressing knees into the body while holding hands, and stretching backs
- Upavistha Konasana—face-to-face, stretching and resting on the back

Twist

- Siddhasana Twist—back to back, opposite side, face-to-face and bind

Back Bends

- Salabhasana—partner back bend; stand up and grab the wrist.

Strength and Inversions

- Navasana—face-to-face with one leg and both
- Sarvangasana and Dandasana with arms up (Sarvangasana—grab the waist; Dandasana—grab the knees or ankles)
- Dandasana and Halasana—support the pose.
- Savasana—heads touch.

Yoga Seniors—Yoga on the Chair

Yoga on the chair is a really popular practice for seniors. It promotes balance and security. A secure practice, it is obtainable for all, leading to a better, healthy lifestyle and opening a brighter state of consciousness. Most of the asana learning in this training can be effective on the chair.

What are important things we need to know as the physical human body ages?

- There is a decrease in muscle mass, heart efficiency, flexibility, cardiovascular health, bone mass/density, or work capacity.
- There is an increase in blood pressure or weight gain.
- Seniors should modify the practice due to concerns of high blood pressure, joint stress, lack of stability, physical ailments, and lack of flexibility.

What can we teach seniors?

- Teach them how to improve their daily health and lifestyle through the practice of yoga.
- Provide useful, practical techniques to be able to maintain mobility in the body.
- Show them how to avoid extending the limbs abruptly or in an unnatural direction.
- Breathe! Cue for full, complete breaths.
- Tell them to move with a slower pace, honor the body, and be kind and gentle to themselves.

Ask and Hints

- Seek permission from doctor to practice—make note of health concerns.
- Provide a longer warm-up.
- Speak loudly and clearly but use a soft tone.
- Use music acceptable to the senior population.
- Use both visual and verbal cueing.
- Repeat the cues for proper alignment for each pose.
- Provide repeated verbal cues and visual demonstrations prior to taking the group into a pose.

- Explain the benefits of the pose.
- Be sensitive to heat and cold. Modify the temperatures, if possible. Suggest layered clothing to help with heat or cold issues.
- Encourage regular participation. Help them to establish a commitment to regular exercise. An attendance roster makes individuals feel needed and wanted.
- A personal phone call when they are absent reinforces the connection to the group. A buddy system encourages class participation.
- Laugh. Have fun! Enjoy the wise. Be encouraging and supportive.
- Avoid complex poses that require a lot of strength. Most seniors are interested in development of functional strength and endurance.
- Repetition of poses is good to help refine and perfect the pose as well as benefit them from the pose.
- Encourage relaxation time (Savasana) at the end of the class. This allows for stress release, learning to relax, muscular resting, and release of tension in the neck, upper back, and cranial areas. Teach meditation.

Keep the instructions simple and safe, knowing that any traditional asana could be transposed to a sitting chair pose.

- Sit on the chair.
- Breathe and center.
- Do neck and shoulders movements.
- Do easy twist—goddess.
- Practice Cat-Cow.
- Stretch front with chest expansion.
- Do leg stretches.
- Implement ankle stretch.
- Do knee stretch.
- SN A—SN B—use a chair to promote balance and security.

- Teach Sun Salutation, considering the breath.
- Do Tadasana.
- Put arms up or forward—Mukha Sirsasana.
- Implement forward fold—Uttanasana; use a chair for support in the fold.
- Execute chest lift—Ardha Uttanasana; use the chair to lengthen the arms and spine; bend the knees if necessary.
- Do forward fold—Uttanasana.
- Put arms up or forward—Mukha Sirsasana or Tadasana.
- Squats—use chair if weakness in the pelvis requires support.
- Lift the ankles and toes.
- Do chair pose—Utkatasana; use chair for support.
- Stretch sides—lateral flexion; use a chair.

- Do Tree—Vrksasana; use a chair.
- Observe Natarajasana—dance pose; stretch the quadriceps.
- Feature kick back—stretch the hamstrings.

- Do Warrior I and II—use a chair, either seated or for support.
- Execute Ardha Chandrasana V—use a chair, seated or for support.
- Do Triangle—Trikonasana; use short chair.
- Use side angle—Parsvakonasana; use short chair.

- Sit on the chair.
- Stretch the quads with launches and a twist.
- Do eagle stretch.
- Open hips.
- Do riding horse.
- Perform meditation.
- Do Savasana.

Yoga for Children

We have already studied the general benefits of the practice of yoga. We know that the practice is good for every single human being as well as for children, the pioneers of the next spiritual civilization.

Why Is Yoga Good for Children?

Yoga brings self-confidence, self-esteem, self-respect, and empathy toward others. The practice of yoga is a unique opportunity to do something without being concerned, whether the right thing is being done or not.

Yoga brings physical force, works all the muscles, and makes them move in different directions and levels. Yoga is a good exercise for children without athletic character. It is right for shy children, those who fear failure and have a tendency to always be late. Yoga activates the nervous system, helps to build energy and stamina, and reduces children's stress levels.

Yoga is a noncompetitive activity. It is a unique activity where children can act with security without the need to win or lose and without judging or feeling threatened by other players. Acceptance is a major part of yoga. Kids learn to accept themselves and understand they are fine the way they are and how they look; there is no need to feel a need to change. They learn to unburden themselves of wanting to be someone else and accept themselves as they are.

Yoga improves internal health; with practice we massage the vital organs and awaken the idea of taking good care of ourselves.

Balance is another vital element of yoga. Yoga can be especially important in developing balance in children. Mental clarity is another benefit; consider, for example, learning to hold the weight of the body on one side. Relatively simple activities such as those increase physical and mental balance, and produce a sensation of self-esteem.

Coordination—children learn to use their bodies differently; they experience and become aware of proper back alignment. Their minds become calm, and this state helps to develop coordination.

Concentration—studies show that the practice of yoga helps children to center and concentrate in school activities; this improves their grades. Yoga helps children to calm their minds and focus in their work; and, at the same time, yoga brings awareness of body parts and functions, an essential part of the practice. Children learn parts of the body easily, including the spine and skeletal structure, articulations, muscles, the cardiovascular system, and so forth. Children learn how to control and manipulate their bodies and enlarge their mobility.

In small children yoga can be used to teach about even the least considered parts of the body. Locate little toes, the jaw, the sternum, and so forth; they learn that all body parts are important and have their function.

Flexibility is obtained though the practice. It helps to prevent injuries in other sports and activities, and children improve their posture as they grow. Children grow in so many ways through the challenges of the practice.

They also learn patience, waiting for their turn with gratitude and respect. Yoga can be a useful tool in teaching manners, compassion, and sharing. In the class we are all the same; we are all friends, and we all grow together as a friendly team. We learn about unity; we are all one—the union—this is yoga.

Warrior Song (with Asana)

I am a strong and proud Warrior (Warrior I).
I move my arms in a cross (cross arms).
I reach forward as the clouds (Warrior II).

My legs go down (Warrior II).
My front arm lifts up (front arm up).
My back arm lengthens down (Ardha Chandrasana V).

I return to home (Warrior II).
I am a very tall warrior (Warrior I).
Don't look at me; I will catch you.

Song for Sun Salutation A

Hands up,
Hands down,
I look to the sky with a very straight back.
I am a strong table.
I lower down slowly to the floor.
I became a snake.
And now I'm a little dog.
I jump and start again.

Song for Sun Salutation B

I sit down in a chair with my hands up,
Hands down.
I look to the sky with a straight spine.
I am a strong table.
I become a snake and afterward a little dog.
The right foot comes forward, and the left leg becomes very strong. I raise my hands and look to the sky—I am a warrior.
Down go my hands.
I am a strong table.
Slowly I lower down.
I became a snake and afterward a little dog.
The left foot comes forward; the right leg becomes very strong. I raise my hands and look to the sky—I am a warrior.
I am a strong table.
I became a snake and afterward a little dog.
Jump, jump. My spine is flat. Down go my hands.
I sit back in my chair and put my arms up.

Teach How to Breathe through Questions

- Do you know where your spine is? (Children answer.)
- Teach the upper, middle, and lower back parts.

- Imagine our backs are like straws.
- Do you know what happens when we drink from a straw? (Children answer.)
- The drink gets into your mouths.
- What will happen if we curve the straw? (Children answer.)
- The drink has problems getting in our mouths.
- Our backs respond exactly the same way. Our backs are like straws that allow all that is good to come in and all that is bad to go out.
- Do you know what things can get in our bodies? (Children answer.)
- There is air (oxygen), food, liquid, vitamins, minerals, and many other healthy things.

Do you know what bad things do to us? One bad thing is carbon dioxide, which we expel every time we exhale. Our lungs don't like it, and they work hard to eliminate it and send it to plants and trees, which do like it and need it. Also we can eliminate mucus and odor, and later we go to the bathroom. When we sit down with bad posture (demonstrate), the straws in our spines collapse, and the good things cannot get inside our bodies easily. Also the bad things cannot go out easily. But when we sit down straight and with good posture, we can breathe deeply and naturally, and we become very healthy. Also, we can use good breathing and posture for other things, such as walking, singing, and teaching these things to other children or even to our parents.

Emotional Control (an example)

Do any of you get mad sometimes? Or maybe feel sad? Or lonely? (Children answer.)

Show Faces of Sadness, Madness, and So Forth

Sometimes when we feel that way, we feel butterflies in our tummies, or we get all chocked up and have trouble talking (and so forth).

You know what I do when this happens to me? I start breathing deeply (show the children how to breathe for ten breaths), and suddenly, when I open my eyes, all these feelings are gone.

So from now on, when you get mad with your brother or sister, don't talk in a mad way to them. Go to your seat, sit down, close your eyes, and breathe deeply ten times; and then you will see what happens. If I am sacred, I breathe. If I am sad, I breathe. If I don't know something, I breathe. I just breathe through everything. When you breathe through your problems, everything becomes much easier; at the same time, you can learn how to sing OM. You must try this, and the next time you can let me know how it went, okay? (Breathe again with the children.)

Remember That They Are Children

- The purpose of yoga is to open the heart, physically and mentally. Keep love and compassion for this practice.
- Every emotion in the world comes from two roots: love or fear. Use love.
- Compare yourself to an animal and perform animal gestures.
- Enjoy your classes, use children's ideas, answer their questions, develop your child-mind, and create games where there is no winner or loser. All their postures are great; as they try to do them, they are doing well. The value is in the effort.
- Don't get too technical and let them be wrong. Show them how to breathe, how to relax, balance, and try to get along with all. This is more important than obtaining a perfect practice.
- The practice is the practice; we can only practice. Yoga is a path for life that brings enlightenment. Everything we learn on our mat we transport into our lives. In yoga there are no trophies. There is no big end. This is just a path, and we are teaching it

to the children. Keep this in mind; you are giving them tools that are really valuable for their lives.

- Flexibility is mental, physical, and spiritual. Yoga brings to children self-esteem, trust, concentration, and consciousness.
- Other teaching techniques include using video in the studio, finding movies (from Disney, for example), developing sequences to follow to songs, and so forth.
- Teaching yoga to children is fun, but at the same time it requires lots of effort and work. You need to be creative, have good energy, and always be ready for their challenges. Observe children out of class and see what they like. Look for new ideas and use different materials. Keep your practice active and maintain your love for children.

Chapter 2

Philosophy of Yoga

The Eight Limbs of Yoga

1. Yama—Abstention
2. Niyama—Observances
3. Asana—Physical Practice of Poses
4. Pranayama—Conscious Breathing
5. Prathayara—Interiorization
6. Dharana—Concentration (Mantra Om)
7. Dhyana—Meditation
8. Samadhi—State of Super-Consciousness

The First and Second Limbs

The Yamas and Niyamas are the first two limbs of yoga. The Yamas are universal moral commandments (natural laws not controlled by the individual), and the Niyamas are rules of personal conduct (controlled by the individual). These are the important rules of conduct a practitioner of yoga should try to follow.

Yama

1. Ahimsa (nonviolence—A, "no"; Himsa—"violence")
   • Loving-kindness to others, gentleness of the use of the body
   • Not blocking or obstructing the flow of nature
   • The yogi realizes that violence rises out of fear, weakness, ignorance, and restlessness.
   • Becoming pure in thoughts, words, and deeds

2. Satya (truthfulness, not to lie)
   - Responding—genuine and authentic to our inner natures
   - Understanding that life is based on truth
   - Having integrity and honesty, being honorable to our truth
   - Not exaggerating or downplaying
   - God is truth, and truth is God.
   - Practicing truthfulness will open the doors to arrangements from God.

3. Asteya (respect for the property of others)
   - No taking what isn't yours (money or goods)
   - Not robbing people of their own experience, ideas, and freedom
   - No desires for other people's positions, qualities, or status
   - Also, the yogi believes that collecting things he or she doesn't use anymore is an act of stealing.
   - Freedom from cravings and desires

4. Brahmacharya (celibacy, sexuality without vice)
   - Relating to others with unconditional love and integrity without selfishness or manipulation
   - Related also to any source of continence
   - Especially in practicing sexual moderation, self-restrain from sexual misconduct

5. Aparigraha (to be free from hoarding)
   - No grasping, nonpossessiveness
   - Not accumulating things beyond what is really necessary and essential
   - Nonattachment to material positions

- A yogi believes hoarding or having greed is just a lack of trust in God and himself or herself to provide for his or her future.
- Make life as simple as possible and train the mind not to feel the loss or lack of anything; trust that everything needed will arrive by itself at the proper time.

The Yamas are rules of behavior nature imposes on humanity. Societies worldwide have created laws with punishments for those who violate these rules.

Niyama

1. Saucha (purity)
   - Purity of body, mind, and soul—this is essential for well-being.
   - Cleanliness, precision, order, and balance
   - Internal and external purification
   - Clear the mind of impure thoughts and emotions such as hatred, anger, lust, greed, delusion, and pride.

2. Santosha (contentment)
   - Contentment, tranquility, and peace are states of mind to be cultivated.
   - Accepting the way things are, finding goodness and beauty in all things
   - As a result of contentment, one gains supreme joy.

3. Tapas (heat, effort to achieve)
   - Tapas is the burning desire for reunion with God, expressed by self-discipline, purification, willpower, austerity, and patience.
   - By the practice of Tapas, the yogi develops strength in the body, mind, and character, obtaining courage and wisdom, integrity, humility, simplicity, and surrender.

4. Svadhyaya (study of the self)
  * Spiritual studies through sacred books, scriptures, chanting, and the Sanskrit
  * Searching for the divine, bringing knowledge and ending with ignorance
  * Implies self-discipline, concentration, and spiritual evolution.

5. Isvara Pranidhana (dedication to God)
  * Willingness to serve the Lord
  * Offering the work to God, tuning with God's will
  * The yogi has learned how to dedicate all actions to God.
  * Surrender to the will of God

Asana

The third limb of yoga is asana. The physical practice of yoga brings power, health, lightness, and agility to the body, mind, and soul. Asana exercises every muscle, all the nerves, glands, and tissues of the body. Asana reduces fatigue, restores energy, and soothes the nervous system. The true importance of the asana is in the interplay of mind and body, and this aids in the transformation of the human being to the maximum extent possible.

The yogi conquers the body with continued practice of asana and transforms this body into a vehicle to guide his or her soul.

The yogi doesn't consider the body his or her property. He or she knows that the universe has loaned him or her this earthly form, and one day it will return to it. What is important is the spirit that resides inside.

With the practice of asana, the yogi is free of physical disorders and mental distractions. The body is a temple of the divine. A yogi isn't negligent; nor does he or she speak ill of his or her body. To the contrary, the yogi cheers up and animates his or her soul.

Pranayama

The fourth limb of yoga is pranayama. *Prana* signifies the life-force, energy, and vitality. *Yama* signifies complete control, extension, and expansion.

The goal is to calm the mind—*"yogas chita vrtti nirodaha."*

The best way to control the mind is through pranayama. The technique of breathing control helps to clean the mind of unwanted thoughts and elevate the body and consciousness to the level of the supreme, the highest of our existence. Pranayama is a consistent prolongation of the following:

- Puraka—inhalation
- Kumbhaka—retention
- Rechaka—exhalation

Prana is the energy used by the soul. It is the force that animates material. Prana exists in everything: food, air, water, and so forth. We begin to control prana through the use of our lungs, and as we practice, we learn to extend this control to all body parts, destroying infirmities and regenerating and invigorating health. Through pranayama we learn to store prana in the third chakra, Manipura, located in the solar plexus. Pranayama and correct diet cure the majority of modern diseases. Little by little it increases our strength, self-control, concentration, and spiritual evolution.

The pranayama breath exercises most familiar and practiced by yogis are Anuloma Viloma, Ujjayi, Kapalbhati, Sitali and Sitakari. An active practice of pranayama liberates the student from daily stress and permits the mind to begin in the correct direction.

Pratyahara

The fifth limb of yoga is interiorization. *Pratyahara* is the state we reach when we have complete control of our senses. The mind is free of desire, and fear is gone. When the power of interiorization has reached the bottom of our consciousness, we feel content.

In this state, the human being can clearly see the three gunas as described in the Ayurveda and Hindu philosophy. The three qualities of nature are the following:

- Sattva: illumination, the light, the good quality that brings clarity and serenity, equilibrium, and effortlessness
- Raja: the quality of activity and movement; the mind is agile and quick.
- Tamas: that which is dark, brings despair, and serves to bring contrast to the light

Dharana

Dharana, the sixth aspect of yoga, is concentration. This is achieved when the body has been seasoned by asana and when the mind has been energized through pranayama. The interiorization, pratyahara, is the direction of thought. In transformation, the student (sadhaka) reaches with dharana, using its power, the power of intense concentration, to attain his or her goal. Without concentration, nothing of consequence can be achieved; concentration in the divine molds and controls the interior energy. In the classic form, the student concentrates on the mantra Aum.

The sound of "Aum" symbolizes the dimension of elongation, breath, and depth (eternal life in the internal, the soul). And with this deep concentration, the student finds freedom from the body, mind, intellect, and ego.

"Om" (Aum) is described in the Vedas as the vibration that forms the essence of total creation.

"Om" (Aum) represents the Hindu trinity of creation, preservation, and destruction—the sound (vibration) of life. This trinity applies to the life of a being as well as the moments of life themselves:

A: creation—the process of generation, our process in the creation of anything; the "creation" is a property that is pure, sacred, and noble.

U: preservation—the action of sustaining and reinforcing the exterior qualities that permit us to remain animated

M: destruction—not a process of loss; destruction dissolves impurities and negativities.

Dhyana

The seventh limb of yoga is dhyana, meditation. Progress on the way of the yogi brings strength to the body and molds the mind, refines the character, and calms the spirit when an elevated level of thought is directed toward God. The illumination of spirit is what liberates the spirit, the soul.

In the state of meditation, sadhaka (the student) discovers the meaning of existence and the will of God. The student finds peace, serenity, and clarity of perception, stability, equilibrium, a lightness, wisdom, and blessing. The grace of complete union permits the sadhaka the deepest feeling of well-being.

Meditation is a simple technique to learn. It is another step on the journey to discover the self. To practice the art of meditation with regularity offers marvelous results; it brings deep mind control over the entire material world.

Samadhi

The last and final limb of yoga is samadhi, where the sadhaka finds unity in all his or her studies and "puts it all together." The state of samadhi is described as "contemplation in the super-conscious state": it is the merging with the mind of God.

A state beyond consciousness, yoga is the union with Brahman, the highest state of the divine.

There are three parts in the makeup of the complete being: body, mind, and soul. One cannot exist without the other two. The most important part is the soul because it is eternal; it never dies. The ignorance of humanity is to forget this teaching, which is so basic and ancient, and to walk on the path without conscience.

When we have a thought, all three parts are moved. The same is true when we feed ourselves. In reality, everything we do impacts the body, mind, and soul. In everything we do, we find an opportunity to contaminate or strengthen our bodies, minds, and souls. The three parts of us can't be separated so as long as we are here on earth; our souls are our energy, our minds are the instruments of our thoughts, and finally our bodies carry the load and operate physically.

Our body is the vehicle God permits us to use to have life in the present. When the soul abandons the body and mind, it goes back to another dimension, to another world. We leave the earth, and we are born in another space, as simply as that. The ones we leave behind are sad to have lost a loved one.

But in the great beyond, they are celebrating our welcome; we are born again. Only the soul survives. Death doesn't exist; life goes on in other forms, other circumstances. The ultimate passage is to arrive at the advanced state of vibration of life and soul, which is the vibration of God, of the divine. That is when we see it all clearly.

Bhakti Yoga, Mantras, Hindu Gods

Bhakti yoga is the yoga of devotion that attracts people with a sense of natural emotive faith. It is the yoga of your heart that establishes through repetition of mantras, chanting. Meditation and enlightenment, the power of love, and the practice of bhakti allow us to understand God as love.

The language of Sanskrit is the language used in yoga, the language of the chants, songs, rituals, and mantras; Sanskrit is the language of energy. It is also the original language of the religions of Hinduism and Buddhism. It is the oldest Indo-European language and the earliest documented. Today it is one of the twenty-two official languages spoken in India.

What does the word *Sanskrit* mean?

Sans, "absolutely"

Krit, "perfect"

The sounds of this language act energetically in the body, and this is how we develop the energy of the mantra in the body.

There are only fifty sounds in Sanskrit, however; the grammar of this language is complex, and the serious student must give much time for full comprehension.

The majority of texts in Sanskrit, those that have been conserved and survive today, were transmitted orally until they were written down in the medieval period in India.

Mantra (Man, "to think"; Tra, "liberation from Samsara")

Samsara—the cycle of life: birth, life, death, and rebirth

Mantras are verses. In Sanskrit they can be chanted or read. The mantras are based in energy, not in comprehension.

When you chant a mantra, you awaken the deepest inner self and connect with a deep state of energy and consciousness; you also obtain power through concentration. The practice of mantra generates endorphins (natural analgesics), lowers the heart rate and blood pressure, and invites you to a state of relaxation and reduction of stress.

Mantra has its origin in the Vedas and is food for the soul.

The Two Forms of Mantra

- Saguna: mantras that invoke the forms of gods. Long mantras have deep meaning.
- Nirguna: mantras that are identified with creation itself and don't invoke personal deities; these are simply sounds—Bija.

What Is Mala, and What Is Japa?

Japa is a meditation that lasts forty days and is a spiritual practice in India. Traditionally, it is performed with a mala (a rosary of 108 beads).

Japa is performed every day at the same place and at the same time.

The mala has the guru bead at the center; it indicates the beginning and end of the rosary. Mala (prayer beads) are used in Hinduism, Buddhism, Islamism, Taoists, Jainism, and so forth.

Popular Forms of God in Hindu Philosophy

Most recognizable is the trilogy: Brahman, Vishnu, and Shiva. The trilogy of Brahman, Vishnu, and Shiva represents the three aspects of the divine, which are creation, preservation, and destruction.

- Brahman (God of creation) instills creativity, overcomes infertility, injects happiness in this world, and aids in the learning process.
- Vishnu (God of preservation) illumines the heart, achieving all success in life, welfare for one's family, and true reverence for life.
- Shiva (God of destruction) destroys ego and false identification, eliminate old habits and attachments, and creates new opportunities.

Other Gods include the following:

Saraswatie is the Goddess of understanding, wisdom, science, art, music, painting, and literature. She is the guardian of the Vedas. Dressed in a white sari, she is also seated on white, representing purity. She is accompanied by a white swan that represents studied thought and intellect. She holds the Vedas, a mala (representing meditation), and plays the vina (a symbol of elegance).

Bija: Om Aim Saraswati Namaha

Lakshmi is the Goddess of wealth, fame, fortune, abundance, and beauty. Her four arms and hands represent the four spiritual virtues: prudence, justice, fortitude, and temperance. She is seated in the lotus position as to be seated on divine truth. She has her hand extended to bless the world.

Bija: Om Shrim Lakshmyai Namaha

Ganesh is the remover of the obstacles so one may reach his or her objectives with success; Ganesh is a symbol of good luck. The enormous size of Ganapati represents the universe, and his curved trunk represents Aum. Ganesh is one of the most popular Gods of India.

Bija: Om Gum Ganapatiye Namah

Durga is the Goddess of protection and destruction. She is a shining Goddess who appears with a lion or tiger. Durga has eight arms, is invincible, and practices mudra with her fingers. Durga comes and shows how to live a life free of fear, with patience and a sense of humor.

Bija: Om Dum Durgaya Namaha

Kirtan is part of the practice of bhakti yoga, the way of devotion of the heart. The roots of Kirtan come from India, where people reunite in the streets to sing, chant, and adore the divinities in unity and happiness; in this way they receive protection and the eternal blessing. Kirtan is a spiritual practice made up of singing, with calls and responses. Today it is known as an enlightened practice that directs a person directly toward the path to liberation.

The mantras and sacred songs purify the mind, open the heart, and awaken the spirit. They create a deep spiritual practice, where one can learn to use time to connect with the divine, the energy of the universe. Kirtan can free the mind of problems and illuminate the deepest feelings of human beings.

Kirtan unifies the community (Sat sang) so all may participate in devotion. It reinforces a collective level and gives the individual a feeling for life. We understand that the practice unifies humanity and cleanses the planet Earth.

"Om Namah Shivay"
Powerful mantra

"I bow to Shiva—supreme reality. Given name to consciousness that dwells in all—Shiva is the name of your own true identity, yourself."

Gayatri Mantra

Aum Bhur Bhuvah Swah
Tat Savitur Varenyam
Bhargo Devasya Dhimahi
Dhiyo Yo Nah Prachodayat

"We salute the sacred sound and present it to the earth, the sky, and the great beyond (heaven). May the splendid glory of the divine Power of Life illuminate our meditation."

Aum—God of the Seven Worlds, guide our minds in the spiritual path. Earth, astral, mental, emotional, creativity, intuition, and absolute truth.

Mahamrityunjaya Mantra (Victory over Death)

Aum Tryambakam Yajamahe
Sugandhim Pusti-Vardhanam
Urvarukam Iva Bandhanan
Mrtyor-Muksiya Mamrtat

This mantra will help you in your health and give long life, peace, liberation, and prosperity

Asato Ma Sad Gamaya

Aum Asato Ma Sad Gamaya
Tamaso Ma Jyotir Gamaya
Mrityorma Amrtam Gamaya
Aum Shanti, Shanti Shantihi

From lies to truth,
From darkness to light,

From death to immortality.
Peace, peace, peace.

Aum Lokha Samasta Sukhino Bhavantu (three times)

"We receive you (we honor you, praise you), for you liberate all beings from poverty and suffering."

Aum

In the Vedas, the oldest writings of India, the mantra Aum is described as the force that creates, the essence of creation. Aum represents the Hindu trinity of creation, preservation, and destruction.

The mantras are so powerful that they can change aspects of one's life, including the people who don't understand the importance of them. It is difficult to understand the deepest meanings of the mantras.

Mantra to Lakshmi

Siddi-Buddhi-Prade Devi
Bhukti-Mukti-Pradayini
Mantra-Murte Sada Devi
Maha-Laksmi Namo 'Stu Te

Lakshmi is the Goddess of fortune and abundance. She is the key to success, intelligence, freedom, and recognition. To recite this mantra is to use mystic syllables to honor and salute the Goddess Lakshmi.

This mantra is for improving your social status, increasing wealth and riches, and promoting one's professional career and personal relationships. In love, it helps to find your matching soul.

Yoga Sutras

The yoga sutras are the sacred books that contain the teachings of yoga.

Patanjali collected and put them together sometime between 500 and 200 BC. It isn't clear whether Patanjali was a single person or a team, since the work of building the sutras took many years, and the work of several authors is involved. However, all we can know from this age comes from legends. It is said that Patanjali was a very evolved and emancipated soul who came to earth of his own will to help and teach the path of yoga to humankind.

The sutras describe the means to recover from the afflictions of the body and fluctuations of the mind, which are the principal obstacles to spiritual evolution.

Legend of the Birth of Patanjali

Lord Vishnu was sitting on his couch. Adidesa, the Lord of the snakes, was absorbed by the presence of the dance of Shiva. Lord Vishnu was so absorbed in the dance of Shiva that his body grew heavier to the point that Adidesa felt Vishnu as a crushing weight on top of him. When Shiva stopped dancing, Vishnu's weight returned to normal, and Adidesa was relieved and amazed at the transformation in Vishnu. Adidesa asked Vishnu to explain what had happened. Vishnu said that Shiva's dancing had been so graceful that his body had begun to vibrate in harmony with Shiva in joy, and this had made him appear heavier and heavier. Adidesa wanted to learn how to dance so she could please Vishnu too.

Seeking a form (a physical body) in which to dance, Adidesa discovered Gonika (a mortal human being), old yogini, who was praying to the sun the wish of having a son to transmit all her knowledge and wisdom. In her ritual Gonika poured water in her cupped hands, closed her eyes, and prayed, expressing the desire of wanting a child.

When she opened her eyes, she found a tiny baby snake floating in the water, asking to be her son. She accepted him, and he transformed into a human being. And that is how Patanjali was born.

What does the name *Patanjali* mean?
Pata, "to fall"

Anjali, "offering" (hands together in prayer position)

Patanjali is not only the author of the yoga sutras; he also wrote grammatical books and chapters of Ayurveda.

- Al Mahabhasya, the classic book of Sanskrit grammar
- Ayurveda, the science of life and good health
- The yoga sutras—directed to the mental and spiritual welfare of the human being

These are the three books that show the integral development of the human being with thoughts, words, and actions.

The effect of yoga is reflected in the actions of the student of yoga. It is a mirror; the yogi observes the reflections of his or her thoughts, mind, and consciousness; and corrects himself or herself, gaining observation toward the interior self.

Sutras

- The yoga sutras are divided into four chapters or four books (Padas).
- There are a total 196 verses or aphorisms (sayings) or sutras. They are precise and profound statements of ideas and knowledge to guide the student (sadhaka) toward wisdom of his or her own authentic nature. The sutras are based in total freedom, beyond common and ordinary comprehension. Through the studies of yoga sutras and devotion, the student obtains supreme knowledge.

The Books of the Sutras:
Samadhi Pada: contemplation, blissful state
Sadhana Pada: practice or discipline
Vibhuti Pada: power, accomplishment
Kaivalya Pada: nature of liberation and transcendental self

Book 1: Samadhi Pada (The Contemplation)

Samadhi Pada is designed for evolved students to allow the maintenance of the mature state of intelligence and wisdom. Samadhi is a guide to discover the source of the consciousness. In the consciousness there exist the three gunas, the three qualities of deep thought:

Sattva: illumination, white
Rajas: vibration, red
Tamas: inertia, black

The second sutra of Samadhi Pada is the conclusion of the descriptions of the meaning of yoga. All instructors of yoga should be familiar with this sutra:

"Yogah Citta Vrtti Nirodhah"

Yogah: union, integration
Citta: conscious movement composed of the following:
        (Mana: mind; Buddhi: intelligence; Ahamkara: ego)
Vrtti: state of mind
Nirodah: control

"Yoga Is Control of the Movement of Consciousness."
"Yoga Is the Restraint of Mental Modification"

In Samadhi Pada we learn that the process of human evolution comes through our internal space.

Unity between ourselves and the physical world is when the mind observes (is awake to the full mental process) the conscious and unconscious and all the activities of the brain combined. All physical activities have their origin in the mind, and all the mind activities have their origin in the soul.

Atman: Soul

Atman has no form; it is separate from the body. It is free, and it is the true essence at the nuclei of the being. Like the mind, the soul doesn't belong to a single specific spot in the body. Atman is latent and exists in all body parts; it feels everything everywhere, and it is universal.

Book 2: Sadhana Pada (Practice, Discipline)

In Sadhana Pada, Patanjali descends to the level less evolved to help and conduct the student to reach absolute liberty. Here appears kriya yoga (action). We find the "first four limbs of yoga." Concepts include the following:

- Ignorance is the source of unhappiness.
- The afflictions of the mind prevent us from the creation of thought, coherency, or imbalance of the body.
- Through purification of the body, senses, and mind, little by little impurities are erased, and the student (sadhaka) reaches a state of serenity.
- Those who don't have ethical discipline or perfect physical health cannot obtain spiritual illumination.
- The body, mind, and spirit cannot be separate while alive on earth; if the body is asleep, the soul follows.
- Asana helps you to get familiar with the body, senses, and intelligence; and it develops attention, sensitivity, and power of concentration.
- Yoga can cure or alleviate our physical, mental, moral, and spiritual sufferings; and perfection is reached. Success is obtained only when the practice is done with love, from the heart with no expectations, and when the dedication is unconditional.

Key Sanskrit concepts by name:

- Yamas—not to become, a fundamental list of laws
- Niyamas—to do, a fundamental list of commandments
- Asana—physical practice
- Pranayama—leads you beyond the senses (sounds, touch, form, or taste)
- Prathayara—withdrawal from the senses, perception, and organic action

Book 3: Vibhuti Pada (Power, Accomplishment)

- A yogi comes to the stage of Vibhuti and has plenty of knowledge of the past, present, and future. He or she is like the functioning of the solar system (in a state of orbiting). The yogi can understand other people's minds. The yogi acquires abilities over natural powers or siddhis.
- The yogi can become supernaturally small, big, more agile, heavy, and so forth. He or she has obtained his or her desires and reached supremacy and sovereignty.
- Vibhuti explains the properties of yoga and its integration (samyama) through concentration, meditation, and profound absorption into the practice. When there is a profound integration between mind, body, and spirit, from the power over nature itself arrives the state of Vibhuti.

Book 4: Kaivalya (Emancipation, Isolation)

- Kaivalya is the fourth pada of the sutras. It is an exposition of the path of detachment, renouncing the objects of this life and thus achieving liberty and a true respect toward them.
- Kaivalya is a positive state, where life and work go together without implication.
- Patanjali teaches us that Kaivalya arrives through birth, mantras through Tapas (intense effort), and Samadhi.

- Yoga allows us to live on the spiritual path; the action of nonyoga leaves us attached to the body and mind, adrift in the world.
- Yoga erases the root of pride in the mind and helps the student to find the source of action, conscious of where the impressions of the past lived (samskara).
- Desire, action, and reaction are estates of the mind. When consciousness becomes pure and stable, the states of mind are eliminated. The yogi becomes perfect and obtains deference from others. The yogi works in the world with detachment; he or she is unaffected. The yogi's mind is pure and without disturbances; he or she arrives at liberation, a finality of experience, total wisdom. This state is blissful and free of base emotions—desire, anger, passion, pride, malice, selfishness, codices, and avarice.
- Kaivalya illuminates the soul of the yogi and all those close to him or her.

First Book: Samadhi (Fifty-One Aphorisms)—Contemplation

1.2 Yogah Citta Vrtti Nirodah—Restriction of the fluctuations of consciousness

1.8 Viparyayah Mithyajñanam Atadrupa—Wrongful knowledge is based in "nonreal" experience. The wrong knowledge generates darkness of the consciousness.

1.12 Abhyasa Vairagyabhyam Tannirodhah—Practice and detachment are the instruments to stop the uncontrolled movements of the consciousness.

1.21 TIVRasamveganam Asannha—The goal is close at hand for those who take the practice in vigor and with intensity.

1.29 Tatah Pratyakcetana Adhigamah Api Antayara—To meditate on God, repeating the sound "Aum," eliminates obstacles that don't allow us to be our own masters of the inner self.

Second Book: Sadhana (Fifty-Five Aphorisms)—Practice

2.1 Tapahsvadyaya Isvarapranidhanani Kryyogah—With a burning desire for the practice, reflect upon and understand the self and sacred texts and surrender in service to God.

2.3 Avidya Asmita Raga Dvesa Abhinivesah Klesah—The five afflictions that imbalance the consciousness are ignorance or lack of wisdom, egocentrism or pride, attachment to pleasure, fear of pain, fear of death, and attachment to life. These hinder personal evolution.

2.8 DUNkha Anusayi Dvesah—Hatred and resentment are related to fear and suffering; unhappiness conducts the mind to the state of hate.

2.16 Heyam Dunhkham Anagatam—The pain and sorrows that still have to arrive can be avoided.

2.46 Stira Sukham Asanam—Asana is corporeal firmness perfect, stability of intelligence, and benevolence of spirit.

Third Book: Vibhuti Pada (Fifty-Six Aphorisms)—Accomplishment

Vibhuti Pada describes a state of continual meditation and relates to the three last aspects of yoga—dharana, dhyana, and samadhi.

Fourth Book: Kaivalya Pada (Forty-Four Aphorisms)—Emancipation, the Absolute Liberty

The Kaivalya teaches that true liberation arrives only when the yogi has reached the goals of life and transcended the gunas. Goals and gunas come back to their natural source, and consciousness is established in its own natural and pure state.

- The sutras may be chanted.

Meditation

Meditation is the seventh limb of yoga—dhyana.

Meditation is the process of returning to your self-interior through your own breath. The world is an imperfect place; we are stressed, worried, and disconnected from our interior. A calm and tranquil mind is a happy mind. Only when the mind is in peace can we find the joy we create with it.

As we meditate, we take some time to spend within ourselves, to establish contact with our breath, centering the attention to the present moment. To communicate with our superior self is to manifest love for the singularity of our own lives. To create quietness within the self is to improve thoughts, feelings, and emotions.

To prepare, do the following:

- Sit in Padmasana, Siddhasana, Virasana, or Baddha Konasana.
- Prepare to relax and do nothing for the next few minutes.
- Sit comfortably, with the spine "straight and tall," while leaving the rest of the body relaxed. Focus on your breathing in and out. Breathe through the nose without stressful effort, softening the sides of the lower rib cage as the abdominal wall.
- Traditional meditation is used for spiritual growth, unfolding inner light, love, and wisdom. We all look for peace and harmony. Regular contact with your inner spirit will catalyze a gradual shift to a higher level of consciousness, centered in the peace, joy, and freedom of your spirit.
- Meditation is the connection between you and God's will.

Meditation 1: Interiorizing the Mind

Sitting with the spine straight, begin to breathe. Focus your attention on the sounds around you. Avoid judgment; just listen to sounds. Perhaps the sounds are of cars going by, birds singing, and so forth. Take account that sounds give your mind a reason to think externally, then return to your breath. Continue to listen without thinking so sounds become only unconscious noise.

Bring your attention to the surface of your body, to your skin—the part that is the most exterior aspect of your body. When your mind becomes distracted or loses focus, return to your skin.

Take into consideration your thoughts; heal and cleanse your thoughts. You are conscious of your thoughts, your skin, and the sounds around you. Fix yourself on how you are observing these three specific spaces and return to feeling your breath. Observe without judgment. All things are equal; there is no desire to change anything. The air rises and falls.

Deepening Consciousness

You can count the length of each breath. When the mind is calm, the breath is calm. Use the sound of "so" on the inhalation and "ham" on the exhalation. Each time the mind leaves its place, you have to return to the presence of the breath.

The more the mind is calmed, the more the breath is calmed—the state of breath and mind becomes one. Introduce a pause between the intervals of inhalation and exhalation.

This is the sacred moment between thoughts; it is here that we establish the dimension between thoughts and the higher consciousness. This is where we awaken the spiritual dimension spontaneously and effortlessly, making the crossing of the conscious with the spirit. We let this happen.

The mind is calm, simply exploring the moment: the moment with enthusiasm, tranquility, self-love, centered in the moment. If your mind is agitated, look to your breathing again. If not, meditate in the presence of your mental peace; feel this moment as a special healing time, a time to clarify and be inspired. We can see how we are wonderful beings in harmony with the universe. In the space of silence, we can refind peace. Continue meditating, seated with the spine comfortably alive and tall.

Gong

Before returning to daily life, take a moment to think about the state to which you want to return. You would like to come back fortified in your interior with confidence, a better sense of humor, and feeling happier, more tolerant, more disciplined, less resistant, and so forth. Put this in your heart, not as a thought but as a feeling; and before you open your eyes, let this new awakening be planted in your heart like a seed that sprouts and grows in power and reason.

Meditation 2: To Heal and Transform

Imagination is more important than knowledge. —Einstein

In this meditation we cultivate the power to perform healing. Images planted with true and pure intentions have the power to transform the mind. We are more form than body. Let this meditation transform you, cleansing and rejuvenating you inside.

Sit up with your spine straight and tall. Take a strong and long inhalation, and exhale the tension of all the musculature of your body, arms, legs, fingers and toes, back, and so forth. Feel the power of the heat throughout your body. Lower your head and relax, feeling the relaxation throughout the body. Repeat three times.

Bring your imagination to the palms of your hands. Feel them with intention; feel the warmth and power of healing that rises from the palms of the hands. The healing energy flows up and toward all directions, clearing and purifying the space near you. It is like magic, the mysterious and delicate part of life.

Move your attention to the base of your spine. Visualize a golden flame in the base of the spinal column, filling this area with power and vitality. Little by little, let this energy—the flame—rise in your spinal column, clearing out any blockage you may have there. This meditation requires an intensity that can be felt; let it rise, revitalizing and cleansing until you sense the golden flame arriving to the center of the brain.

Absorb the flame that has arrived in your medulla (the center of the brain) and let it become a glowing ball of powerful golden energy. Let it move and feel it traveling in your head—left, right, up, and down—with a smooth calming motion of cleansing, healing, relaxing and realigning as it goes as if it were a magical and miraculous ball of pure energy, rejuvenating each cell. If you have trouble moving the ball in a determined direction in a specific area, this indicates a blockage or disequilibrium. Continue with intensity, smoothly melting away the blockage, noting that it is becoming easier and easier each time.

Let the glowing ball descend into the core of the body to the deep interior; pass it into the pelvic region and hips. Gently let it rise again to the base of the skull, allowing it to pass through new passages it hasn't touched before. Let it descend again; take the time to feel the new sensation in your body, a brilliant state of health and peace throughout the body—a profound relaxation. You are conscious, alert to the exterior of your body like an aura, like the shell of an egg. Meditate on this aura, forget your body, and feel that your skin is the foundation of this aura, the base surface.

Let the mind be absorbed in this moment. Feel the sensation that you are centered in infinity of inspiration, meditation, and light. If a distraction appears, return to your respiration and meditate again on this state, contacting your spirit.

Gong

Bring your attention to your breath and your body. Let your head drop gently forward and then raise it a little. Open your eyes so they are halfway open and then open all the way.

Look at yourself as part of the infinite sensation you have just experienced.

Meditation 3: Happiness, Discovering Your Heart

The experience of happiness is always present in the spiritual heart that resides in the center of the chest.

This meditation will help you to awaken the conscious heart, erasing sadness and pains, awakening joy, and eliminating suffering. It raises the consciousness to allow more joy in, to let go of old ideas and attachments, and to invite the light of truth for the well-being of the heart.

Sitting tall with the legs crossed, begin to feel your physical body as its parts—head, shoulders, back, torso, legs, arms, hands, and feet. Feel your musculature; sense what is tense, what is relaxed, cold, warm, and so forth. Observe how you can feel your body. What is it that your body is telling you?

Conduct your attention to the top of your head, to the seventh chakra. Take a moment to consider the extraordinary power of the universe to heal and cleanse.

On the next inhalation, absorb the light of the universe through your corona. Exhale and allow the light you feel to comfortably settle deeply in the heart.

On the next inhalation, collect all the stress, negativity, pain, suffering, and the heaviness. Visualize these things leaving the heart.

On the next exhalation, send all these negative emotions away; blow them to the outside.

Practice this exercise several times; when inhaling, we take in vibrations of love. Upon the exhalation, we place them in our heart. On the inhalation, gather all the negative vibrations and upon the exhalation cast them out to the other side of the universe. This practice is easiest and most effective when the breath is easy and smooth. The cycle of eliminating the darkness and negativity and replacing it with a feeling of positive light helps the spirit to be happy and content. You may use this mantra:

Sat (inhale)
Yam (exhale)

Let your breath be tranquil and easy, not forced. The light of happiness resides in your heart. Meditate on this state; meditate with the intention of discovering a little more, this light and power that exist in the self, interior, in the center of the chest. Your mind isn't tired or distracted; it is fixed on the heart. Continue meditating in the abundance of joy, peace, and light.

Gong

Open your eyes and enjoy.

Meditation 4: Erasing the Past

Sit in your base and align the spine with the proposition that you want to know who you are.

Feel the essence of who you are; breathe and be centered in your interior, seeking the center and the past. Seek for the key to transformation. Look back on your life and note what remarkable things have been happening to you—some negative things and others positive. Consider it all a part of the past. This is the base of your life; these days, these experiences are with you. Thanks to these experiences, you are who you are today.

Take note of the instructions you have recorded in your memory, which you use to analyze as good or bad what to hold onto and what to cast off, for you to be who you are.

Fear doesn't allow you to go forward; the resistance to change is the basis for suffering. You are the incarnation of the memories of the past. You are living your life based on a fraction of your memories.

When there is pain, it's the memory of pain. When there is happiness, it is the memory of happiness. If you have problems now, surely they are founded on, or related to, limitations of your parents. Have you looked at your life in these simple terms? This is how your life has been limited since a very young age.

The five categories of the state of mind are interpretations of the mind of a child—everything happening is invoked from a memory of the past; the present is a reaction and can be appreciated as part of a vibration. This reaction forms your habits and is your master until you comprehend it, can direct it, and run with it. Until then it continues its hold on you.

Go back to your childhood; remember your brothers and sisters, parents, the schools, the teachers, and the good and bad times. Then look forward into adolescence; recall the frustrations and the new sensations. Follow the life-force; abandon the grip of these memories and permit more and more energy to flow into your body without restriction. You arrive at twenty years old and keep going until you reach the present; continue investigating your life right up to the present moment. Bring the true richness of who you are into the presence of your life and your actual situation.

Begin to feel the force of your life, the life-force. Sense the first chakra, the second, third, fourth, fifth, sixth, and finally the seventh. The energy is running through your body in the center of your spine, integrating all the experiences of the past.

Bring your consciousness to your first aura, approximately one centimeter beyond the surface of your skin. Extend your consciousness out to the second layer of aura; there are no barriers. Continue in the third, the fourth, until you reach the fifth aura, about one meter more until your body forms in a golden globe. This is you—big, wide, large, enormous, and infinite. This is you; this is your reality.

This is who you are in the human form, with your thoughts, loves, pains, and truth. This is the vehicle you have created for your life. You are this band of light, and in it you reside, a marvelous being. Feel the essence of these cells because they form who you are, the interior of who you are. With this exercise you move farther from who you are in the three dimensions.

Sit in the depth of this experience, breathing in the future and letting go of the past, abandoning past wounds. There is a brilliant future that awaits you. By giving up the past and its pains, you seek a future without suffering. Breathing out a past, freeing up from attachment to suffering without giving it note, casting off this master to let it fall back to the stones from which it came, breathing in the future and allowing the eternity of your being to come to its feet. In this magic place where life resides, all is alive; here you realize and encounter the truth. Everything converges at the same place. Love appears, and the spirit expands to encompass the universe and eternal life.

- First Chakra—Lam—Red—Earth
- Second Chakra—Vam—Orange—Water
- Third Chakra—Ram—Yellow—Fire
- Fourth Chakra—Yam—Green—Air
- Fifth Chakra—Ham—Blue—Sound
- Sixth Chakra—Om—Violet—Light
- Seventh Chakra—All Sounds and Colors

Meditation 5: Sensation in the Body

Seated in a comfortable position for meditation, feel the sensations of the body, those that normally don't hold your attention. Circulate mentally through the body, beginning with the toes, feet and legs, knees, thighs, buttocks, waist, stomach, chest, shoulders, arms and elbows, forearms, wrists, hands, fingers, throat, chin, lips, tongue, nose, cheeks, ears, eyes, forehead, and so forth.

Don't linger more than five seconds on each part of the body. Repeat this exercise; after twenty minutes, go back again and feel the sensation of finding each part of the body. This exercise gives you a profound relaxation for your body. The biggest enemy of the body is nervous tension, living too much in the head with little sensation of the body. We must be in the present at all times, forgetting about the past and future. One must learn this technique to awaken the interior senses.

Connect with your sensations again, feeling the parts of your body and organs.

Strengthen your interior with these sensations. If the mind is distracted, go back to the sensations; seek a way to maintain the state of being alert from the sensations in the body. The sensation of integrity will be with you; meditate on it for a few minutes. Observe the silence, meditate on it, look for the silence, and find the success in it. Feel content within this space of silence.

Gong

Little by little, come out of this meditation. Lower the head, open your eyes, and come back to the light of day.

Chapter 3

Physical and Energetic Anatomy

Muladhara

First Chakra

Perseverance
Element—Earth
Color—Red
Sound—Lam
Force—Gravity
Truth—We Are All One

- Location: base of the pelvis
- Lives: mental and emotional foundation
- Source: good health, confidence in life, identity, security, friendship
- Offers: facility to relax, stability, prosperity, and patience
- Physiologically: it connects with family, beliefs, inherited traditions, identity, home situations, and tribal culture.
- Symbolically: it needs to find order and structure, organization, and discipline.
- Deficiency: general bad health, disconnection of the body/mind. Low weight—anorexia, anxiety, and depression, lack of discipline or order, general disorganization.
- Excess: obesity, difficulty in losing weight, overeating, gluttony, fatigue, fear of change, oversecurity

- Equilibrium: great health, vitality, being in comfort with your body, feeling confident, knowing how to relax, finding security and freedom of your actions, having stability in your path
- Illnesses that develop in Muladhara: related to spinal column, rectum, large intestine, immune system, legs, hips, feet, bones and teeth, malfunction of intestines, lumbar pain, constipation or diarrhea, problems in bones, multiple personality, alcoholism, and drugs addictions.

Best Asana
Physical and Spiritual Desires
All Standing Poses, Forward Folds, Hip Openers, Balasana
Birth, Family/Ancestors, Community and Social, Profession

Swadhistana

Second Chakra

Gratification
Element—Water
Color—Orange
Sound—Vam
Force—Opposition
Truth—To Honor All Things

- Location: underneath the navel
- Lives: emotions, feelings, sensations, sexual energy
- Source: maintain relationships with other people, feeling the essence of human being.
- Offers: pleasure, positive attitude open to change of life, gratitude
- Psychologically: it connects with the relation between reactions and responses.
- Symbolically: it needs to find joy and pleasure in the actions.

- Deficiency: social problems, inability to enjoy, fear of change, lack of desire and passion, fear of sex
- Excess: sexual addiction, manipulative seduction, exceedingly strong emotions, hysteria, bipolar, change of humor
- Equilibrium: good relation with others, emotional intelligence, ability to experience pleasure and provide for oneself and others, facility to adapt to new changes, facility to let go of the past
- Illnesses that develop in Swadhistana: related directly to sexual organs, large intestine, lower vertebra, pelvis, hips, circulatory system, genitals and testicles, appendix, kidneys, uterus, and prostate
- Malfunction manifested on brittle bones, reproductive disorders, gallbladder, urinary tract problems, menstrual difficulties, sexual dysfunctions, impotence, lower back pain, knee problems, loss of flexibility, loss of appetite for food, sex, and life

Best Asana
Confidence and Commitment
Standing Positions, Forward Folds, Hip Openers, Yoga Mudrasana
Pleasure, Abundance, Sexuality, Well-Being

Manipura

Third Chakra

Definition
Element—Fire
Color—Yellow
Sound—Ram
Force—Combustion
Truth—Self-Honor

- Location: solar plexus

- Lives: personal power, autonomy, identity, self-esteem, self-respect, confidence
- Source: control of energy, responsibility, fears, personal honor
- Offers: ability to make decisions, egocentrism personality, self-recognition
- Psychologically: relates to the relationship with others and oneself
- Symbolically: has the key to process any physical and emotional experience
- Deficiency: sense of guilt, shame, embarrassment, traumatic experiences, lack of energy and will, easy manipulation, sense of blaming others, low immune system, fear of punishment, inherited emotional issues, lack of discipline, envy of others, criticism
- Excess: creates aggressive behavior, domination, control of all situations, competition, ambition, obstinacy, arrogance, hyperactivity
- Equilibrium: good and healthy sense of humor, self-confidence, spontaneity, playfulness, ability to help others, good function of digestive track, respect for own life, right to act, right to live in freedom
- Illnesses that develop in Manipura: related to the health of stomach, pancreas, gallbladder, adrenal system, digestive track, metabolic organs, large intestine, liver, kidneys, and abdominal muscles. Malfunctions are manifested in low self-esteem, fear, blame, eating disorders, digestive problems, diabetes, muscular spasm, chronic fatigue, hypertension, stomach ulcers, arthritis, and hepatitis.

Best Asana
Courage
Chakravakasana, Downward Facing Dog, Back Bends, Twists
Honor and Values, Self–Esteem, Confidence, Freedom

Anahata

Fourth Chakra

Acceptance
Element—Air
Color—Green
Sound—Yam
Force—Equilibrium
Truth—Love

- Location: in the chest, heart area
- Lives: love, compassion, and hope
- Source: worries, deep thoughts, forgiveness
- Offers: inner peace and tranquility, identification with others
- Psychologically: related to repression of love, hatred, resentment, passion, pain, self-love, and bitterness
- Symbolically: the fourth chakra overcomes emotional blocks.
- Deficiency: trauma, abuse, rejection, feeling abandoned and lost, criticism, abuse of other chakras, cold, and feeling threatened, hurting others. Deficiencies in the fourth chakra leave us antisocial, self-absorbed in negative, selfish ways, intolerant, jealous, alone, afraid of relationship and intimacy, and a lack of empathy.
- Excess: conditional love, imbalance of love, sudden change of feelings
- Equilibrium: compassion, empathy, self-esteem, altruism, peace, balance, healthy immune system. This chakra gives us our emotional perception; it is what determines the quality of our lives more than our mental perception, the flame of our hearts.
- Illnesses that develop in Anahata—related to the physical workings of the heart and circulatory system, breast and rib cage, the lungs, diaphragm, shoulders, arms, legs, neck, and throat, including the glands in these regions. Malfunction of

heart, lungs, diseases, cancer, chest pains, asthma and general lack of breath, pneumonia, circulation problems, and allergies.

Best Asana
Hope and Effort
All Back Bends
Unity, Humanity, Peace, Love, Purity, Innocence

Vishuddha

Fifth Chakra

Expression
Element—Sound
Sound—Ham
Color—Blue
Force—Resonance
Truth—Surrender to the Divine Will

- Location: neck and throat
- Lives: "natural sound." It is the seat of our self-expression, the way to positive action, voice and speech, and creativity.
- Source: harmony with self
- Offers: vibration for peace and joy.
- Psychologically: It is tied to our physical resistance. It is connected with the choices we make in our lives.
- Symbolically: it represents the maturing of the will.
- Deficiency: fear to speak and express oneself, difficulty of expressing one's feelings, timidity, deafness, poor vocal skills (like mumbling speech), and poor sense of hearing
- Excess: speaking too much, being defensive in speech, having a domineering voice, interrupting others

- Equilibrium: a resonant, clear voice; being a good listener; clear verbal communication, with good rhythm; intonation; direction; and a creative life are signs of a healthy fifth chakra.
- Illnesses that develop in Vishuddha: trauma, verbal abuse, lies, constant yelling, authoritarian parenting, overly dependent children
- Disorders with Vishuddha chakra are associated with the functioning of the trachea, esophagus, thyroid gland, cervical portion of the spine, the neck muscles, as well as the jaw, mouth and teeth, shoulders, arms and hands, vocal cords, and ears.

Best Asana
Sweetness, Calmness of Voice, Surrender to the Divine
All Asana That Include Jalandhara Bandha: Sarvangasana, Halasana, Setu Bandhasana, and So Forth
Communication, Integrity, Truth, Will, Creativity

Ajna

Sixth Chakra

Reflection
Element—Light
Color—Indigo
Sound—Om
Force—Sight
Truth—The Quest for Truth

- Location: forehead, "the third eye," the spiritual eye between the eyebrows
- Live: imagination, visualization, dreams, and visions
- Source: power to absorb light, intuition
- Offers: emotional intelligence

- Psychologically: the result of what we know and believe to be the truth
- Symbolically: represents the seat of wisdom, emotional intelligence
- Deficiency: vision problems, memory loss, inability to grasp the future or imagine alternatives, general lack of imagination, difficulty to visualize, inability to remember dreams
- Excess: hallucinations, delusions, obsessions, inability to concentrate from overactive and scattered thinking, nightmares
- Equilibrium: intuition, perception, imagination, clarity and range of memory, the ability to recall and resolve issue of dreaming, and the basic physical quality of good eyesight. Wisdom is the hallmark of the sixth chakra in equilibrium.
- Illnesses that develop in Ajna: They range from the common headache to vision problems, to depression and insanity, and to blindness.
- We connect with the physical world through our body's physical systems. These include our brain, neurological system, pituitary, our external sense organs, eyes, nose, and so forth.

Best Asana
Physical and Spiritual Knowledge
Yoga Mudra and All Meditation Poses
Wisdom, Knowledge, Imagination

Sahasrara

Seventh Chakra

Knowledge and Wisdom
Element, Thought
Color—Violet
Sounds—All

Force—Consciousness
Truth—Living in the Present

- Location: top of the crown of the head, two to three inches above top of the head
- Lives: connection between our physical selves and the infinite universe
- Source: thoughts with which we reach the infinite love and God
- Offers: the light, values; courage and humility, faith, inspiration, spirituality, and devotion
- Psychologically: generates devotion, inspiration, and prophetic thoughts, transcendent ideas, and prana. This energy is stimulated; flows through songs, mantra, and meditation; and also protects us.
- Symbolically: it contains the purest form of energy and grace. The seventh chakra is the center for our interior spirit, vision, intuition, and consciousness. This is a mystic concept, a dimension for relating to God.
- Deficiency: cynicism about the existence of the spirit, learning disorders, apathy, rigid belief systems
- Excess: confusion in general, hyperintellectualism, spiritual addiction, and confusion about the connection of the mind and body with spirit
- Equilibrium: ability to perceive, analyze, assimilate information, intelligence, alertness, open mind, spiritual transcendence, wisdom, and abundant knowledge
- Illnesses that develop in Sahasrara: catastrophic and mental illness including coma, brain tumors, amnesia, and loss of mind

Best Asana
Physical and Spiritual Knowledge
Yoga Mudra, All Meditation Poses
Beauty, Serenity, Unity
Energetic Anatomy

The Three Gunas

According to Hindu philosophy, the gunas are the principal qualities of nature. These qualities are of three types: sattva, rajas, and tamas.

These qualities exist in all things to varying degrees and combinations, including human beings. The gunas determine the nature of the individual—his or her actions, behavior, attitudes, and attractions to the things of this world.

- When sattva predominates, illumination and knowledge radiate from a person.
- When rajas predominates, desire for material wealth and egotism appears.
- When tamas predominates, the results are darkness, disillusionment, inactivity, and depression.

We play within these three conditions.

As the gunas are part of nature; food can also be sattvic, rajasic or tamasic.

The gunas, regardless of being sattva, raja, or tamas, are a part of nature—a nature of which we are a part. We are responsible for our dreams, aspirations, and sufferings. Understanding the immutable properties of the gunas is a very basic concept for the yogi.

The Sattvic Diet of the Yogi

The yogi's diet is a vegetarian one consisting of foods that are pure, simple, and natural. These foods are easy to digest, and they generate good health and well-being. They are simple, clean, and unprocessed sources of nutrition that are easy for the body to digest and assimilate.

Foods that are essential and basic for maintaining stable and richness of health consist of the following:

- Cereals: wheat, rice, oats, millet, barley, quinoa, and so forth
- Legumes: lentils, beans, soy, chick peas, and so forth

- Vegetables
- Fruits and nuts
- Fermented products: yogurt, kefir, choucroute, pickles, and so forth
- Seeds: sesame, pumpkin, sunflower, and so forth
- Proteins: eggs, seitan (wheat), tofu (soy), cheese, and so forth
- Minerals, vitamins, and enzymes (found in all the above and in raw food)
- Fats: vegetable oils, olive, sesame, sunflower, and so forth

Positive Changes in Diets

Substitute artificial foods with natural and vitalizing foods.

Natural foods are ones that have been growing in fertile soils, and they are consumed in their natural state without taking away or adding anything else. They are alive and rich in prana. Organic fruits and vegetables have more vitamins, minerals, and enzymes; and they offer a stronger potential to prevent and cure ailments in the body. Packaged foods or manipulated foods have colorants, conservatives, oxidants, and pesticides.

- It is important as yogis to start changing habits and introducing refined foods in the place of whole foods. Refined foods pass through a transformation in which they lose protein, good fats, fibers, vitamins, mineral salts, and oligoelements.
- Take in more raw foods than cooked foods. Cooking destroys enzymes, vitamins, and dissolved minerals.
- Take in more vegetable food sources than animal products. Proteins from some vegetables (almonds, sesame seeds, soy, peanuts, sunflower seeds, pumpkin seeds, and so forth) are stronger than animal sources.
- Avoid bad fats (solid fats), which are not like good fats (liquid, unsaturated fats).
- Avoid eating too much protein. Excess of protein causes autotoxemia, acidification, uric acid, putrefaction in the

intestines, and imbalances in the mineral system (meat contains more phosphorous than calcium). It activates series illness as arthritis, osteoporosis, cardiovascular problems, cancer, Alzheimer's, and so forth.

- Consume quality good fats such as virgin vegetable oils. Avoid processed margarines and butters.
- Avoid too much salt (maximum: one to two grams per day), sea salt, or Himalayan salt.
- Good sweeteners include whole fruits, honey, molasses, agave syrup, quality maple syrup, and so forth.
- Avoid white sugar.

There is a "food cycle" in nature, often simply called the "cycle" or the "food chain." The sun is the basis for all energy, all life on earth, and it directly feeds the earth and its plant life.

Foodstuffs that receive light directly from the sun are called primary foods, and they have the highest nutritional quality. These are the natural foods—fruits and berries, vegetables, legumes, cereals, seeds, and nuts. They provide varying levels of essential nutrition. Proteins from these foodstuffs, when they reach the stomach, are easily assimilated into the body.

Secondary foodstuffs come from the flesh of animals. These animals have fed on primary foods. The secondary foods are more difficult to digest and have less metabolic value when eaten.

Many people (vegetarians and meat eaters alike) worry that they're not getting enough protein; however, they don't recognize other factors. The quality of the protein is more important than simple quantity of the protein. Dairy, legumes, nuts, and seeds can provide the vegetarian with sufficient high-quality proteins.

The saying "Eat to live, don't live to eat" points us toward the concept that we eat food to maintain our bodies. The energy, the force of life, however, comes from prana, the vital energy. This helps us to understand why the ideal diet for the yogi is a simple diet of fresh foods, a diet in which the foods themselves are full of prana.

The diet of an authentic yogi is even more select. The yogi is aware of the effect that food and eating habits have on the mind and astral body. The yogi prefers foods that aren't overly stimulating, foods that maintain physical calm and an alert intellect.

The yogi committed to the path of yoga avoids eating meat, fish, eggs, onions, garlic, tea, coffee, alcohol, and drugs. Onions and garlic are also considered pungent foods that aren't easily eaten or digested.

Any change in diet a person chooses to make in life (and this can be especially true for some beginners on the path of yoga) should be undertaken gradually.

Abandoning animal proteins, for example, means replacing these with a large quantity of vegetables and derivatives of soy products (tamari, miso, tofu, tempe), nuts, and seeds until this transformation is complete (until the animal proteins are eliminated and the metabolism responds completely). The yogi diet will help you achieve and maintain a wonderful level of health, mental power, and serenity.

The diet of the yogi is a sattvic diet. The sattvic diet permits a clarity and tranquility of the mind that is favorable for the development of spiritual growth. It is a diet that is fresh, good tasting, and enjoyable. The sattvic diet includes basically all the fruits, seeds, nuts, green leafy vegetables, soy products, whole cereals, honey, clean water, and milk. Today, in these times of processed foods and global pollution, only natural, organic foods are considered sattvic. Frozen or canned vegetables, for example, are not considered sattvic.

Rajasic foods may feed the body, but they are stimulating and lead to a tiring and worn-down state of the body and mind. Rajasic foods unbalance the mental equilibrium, and for this reason, the yogi tends to avoid them. Rajasic foods include heavily seasoned cooked foods and stimulants such as coffee, tea, chocolate, eggs, garlic, onions, meats, fish, and all forms of processed foods. These foods should be avoided by anyone seeking peace of mind, but on the other hand, those seeking a life of activity and physical stimulation may choose these foods.

Tamasic foods are to be avoided. They make you fat and put you to sleep; they provide no benefit. They include alcohol as well as old and heavy foods, artificial drinks, and sodas. Overeating is considered a tamasic activity. According to traditional teachings, the stomach should be half full with healthy foods and one-quarter full with water, and the remaining quarter should be empty.

The "nature" of food can change. Heating (cooking) changes the nature of food. The cereals become sattvic only after they have been cooked. Honey becomes tamasic when cooked.

The nature of foods can also change when they are combined with other foods or spices or stored for long periods.

Cultivate the following habits:

- We eat only when we are hungry; it is very important to purify the organism with semifasting—liberating the organs of toxicity, helping them to rest, and healing the digesting organs.
- Semifasting with fruits is the most effective and inoffensive way to recover and maintain health.
- Eat slowly; sit down to eat in a relaxing manner.
- It is better to eat small and varying portions than big and regular, boring amounts of food. It is also important to respect the hours for taking nutrition—eating late at night should be avoided. Nourishment should be prepared fresh and eaten with attention, respect, and gratitude. Food should be tasted and savored, chewed slowly and thoroughly, and prepared and served with love and consciousness.

Ayurveda, Energetic Anatomy

The word *Ayurveda* derives from the ancient language of India, Sanskrit, and signifies "the Knowledge of Life." It is an ancient alternative medicine system referred to by the Hindu ancient terms as the five fundamental states of nature. These are earth, water, air, fire, and space, which compose the universe as the human body.

The science of Ayurveda is found in the Vedas, the ancient books of Hindu wisdom. More than sixty preparations of herbs have been found written in the first Vedas (2,500 BC). The Vedas include solutions to combat illness and pain, and it shows how to overcome obstacles in life.

The Ayurveda is considered much more a medical guide; in reality the Ayurveda is the science of life, of the holistic path, of holistic medicine. It is a guide to longevity, a system of complete care, and a cure for the whole person, physical as well as mental.

Ayurveda continues to be a fountain of light to conserve, maintain, and renovate health and well-being. The basic concept of this science is that each person has the capacity to take control of his or her own self-evolution, including the capacity to cure himself or herself when illness (disequilibrium) strikes.

According to the Ayurveda, there are many forms of energy essentially in all things in varying combinations. These energies make up the universe. These combinations of energy are responsible for life in the universe in the fundamental states of being. We encounter these beings in the process of growth, development, maintenance, and deterioration. Considering that we are talking about energy and the flow of energy, it follows that our acts, our actions, contribute to the direction these processes are going.

Ayurveda describes seven types of tissues of the body, known as plasma, blood, flesh, adipose (body fat), bones, marrow (tissues inside bones), nervous system, and reproductive system (semen, female cells).

In Ayurveda the principal characteristics that distinguish this science are the doshas. The Ayurveda defines the doshas (the types of energetic forces) into three categories that control the activities of the body:

- Vata: air and space. Vata is responsible for the vital functions ranging from the intestines and lumbar region to bones and skin.
- Pitta; fire and water. Pitta is the energy of the process of transforming the nutrients in food to feed the body.
- Kapha: water and earth. Its mission is growth and the creation and addition of tissue, unit by unit, cell by cell.

When the three doshas are in perfect harmony and functioning in equilibrium, good health and well-being are seen in the individual.

When these three energies fall out of equilibrium, we have a problem or disturbance. The science of Ayurveda is to maintain health and prevent disease.

The three energies, the doshas, go out of equilibrium from a basic, easy-to-understand, phenomenon such as inadequate diet, unhealthy surroundings, stress, trauma, wounds, and so forth—in short, the origins of bad health.

Ayurveda focuses on the practice of yoga and meditation.

The Nadis

Once we have studied and understood the concept of the chakras—described as energetic points of being—we can look at nadis. The nadis are the interior channels of the body through which energy flows. There are three principal nadis: Ida, Pingala, and Sushumna.

The word *nadi* means the following: nada, "canal"; di, "fluid."

The nadis are the channels that transport prana, the energy of life.

Pranayama is the technique of breathing, the act to bring a flow of energy through the body. This flow on the mystic plane acts through and serves to purify and develop the channels (the nadis) themselves. On the mystic plane, the flow of this energy through this system acts to awaken kundalini.

- Ida is the "left" channel, the "white" channel. It is feminine, cold, and associated with the light of the moon. In terms of separate "body and mind," it controls the mind. It originates in Muladhara and ends in the left nostril. Each nadi is associated with a river; ida is related to the Ganges River.
- Pingala is the "right" channel, the "red" channel. It is masculine, hot, and associated with sunlight; it controls the body. Pingala begins in Muladhara and ends in the right nostril. It is related to the Yamuna River
- Sushumna is the central channel that follows the spinal column. Sushumna begins in Muladhara and ends in Sahasrara. The energy of kundalini travels in the Sushumna nadi. The river

associated with Sushumna is the Saraswati. The Saraswati River valley in India was the birthplace of Indian culture; the river itself no longer exists, but the valley is now occupied by the Yamuna and the Ganges.

Awakening Kundalini

Kundalini in Sanskrit is translated as "coiled" and is symbolically represented by a goddess or a sleeping serpent. Located in the root of Muladhara, kundalini follows through the energy channel of Sushumna related to consciousness.

The first sign in the awakening of kundalini is a physical, relaxed comfort in the pelvic region where Muladhara resides.—the vibration of the awakening kundalini. This feeling, nurtured by continuing yoga practice, lasts for days.

Later, this relaxed comfort will be felt to rise in the lower spine, and kundalini is said to be seated in reflection. Again, if the process is developing, this sensation will last a number of days. The relaxed feeling will have a sensation said to be like the peacefully swirling eddies in a flowing river; the power begins flowing up the channel of Sushumna in the spinal cord.

The pranic current is flowing and rising, filling all the cells of the body. The body tingles. During this time, there is a unique joy felt physically in the body. As the bandhas become fully aligned, the Sushumna channel is completely cleared of impurities (diet and pranayama exercises are fundamental to this process), and the body begins to experience the tingling as a sustained sense of well-being. To fully awaken kundalini requires several years of sustained practice and a clean diet. Symbolically, a serpent resides in Muladhara, curled up in three coils. The serpent lies sleeping in the base of Muladhara with the kundalini, the sacred energy, in its mouth. waiting to be awakened.

The objective of kundalini yoga style is to wake up the kundalini so it can begin its journey. Breathing exercises and the circulation of energy through Ida and Pingala, the energetic side channels, awaken the force of kundalini that rises through Sushumna, energizing the seven chakra. From the base of Muladhara, Ida and Pingala spiral upward, crossing at each chakra until they unite at the sixth chakra, the "third eye," where they reunite with Sushumna.

Suggestions for a Purer Life

Optimum good health can be considered a state in which the life-force is plentiful in all three levels of existence; physical, mental, and spiritual. The human being is healthy when the cells are healthy, when the tissues the cells form are healthy, when the organs formed of the tissues are healthy, and when the systems of the body—the systems of the organs—are healthy. This is the description of a healthy organism, and the human being is an organism.

The health of a cell depends on the quality of the nutrients that feed it, the ability of the cell to assimilate those nutrients, and the power of the cell to cast off waste residues from the process.

Toxins enter the body through different methods, including penetration through the skin and the circulatory system. Toxins can enter from the air through the lungs or from food or water through the digestive system.

Every day stress affects the nervous and endocrine systems. If we don't give the cells what they need, and if they retain toxins, our health is compromised.

Indications of Toxicity in the Body

The symptoms of toxicity in the body are well known and generally straightforward to observe. They may include loss of will, appetite, and sexual desire as well as insomnia, chronic fatigue, depression, mood shifts, sleeping disorders, obvious outward signs of a bad condition such as obesity, or signs of ailments and pain, eruption of the skin, headache, anxiety, and so forth.

Toxins exist in all parts of the world in which we live: in the air, water, food, and artificial lighting; in containers for food, in preparation of food, in soaps and shampoos, and in our own behaviors, including smoking, drugs, stress, bad habits, and so forth.

It's impossible to live completely free of toxins.

The change, the solution, or the alternative is living with intention and purpose, actively having desire to purify body, mind, and spirit. Intentionally start changing habits that lead to the accumulation of toxins and open to the healing process and forgiveness. Investigate your body and your behavior. Locate and admit the need for changes and make them. In this way you become a reflection of the yogi way, a guiding light for others.

Changes

Here are some activities to avoid:

- Drinking water from the tap
- Eating canned or packaged foods
- Eating red meat
- Using stimulants such as tobacco and caffeine
- Being overweight or underweight
- Staying for long periods under artificial light
- Doing exercises of hyperactivity
- Working for many continuous hours
- Watching violent TV programs and movies
- Holding in anger
- Being impatient
- Lacking sleep
- Being pessimistic
- Focusing on personal limitations
- Thinking about what you don't have
- Having thoughts of desperation and doubt
- Feeling disconnected from others
- Desiring control
- Playing the victim or blaming bad luck
- Indulging in spending sprees

- Having judgment, prejudice, or conditional love
- Working in a state of fear or doubt

Here are some activities to make habits in your life:

- Drinking plenty of filtered and purified water
- Eating fresh and organic foods
- Eating easily digested protein
- Using herbal medicines and herbal teas
- Maintaining your weight
- Working in natural light
- Listening to soothing music and natural peaceful sounds
- Practicing yoga, walking, and swimming
- Forgiving others and yourself for not being perfect
- Having confidence that each moment is perfect for your life
- Sleeping deeply
- Being optimistic and positive
- Being open to new possibilities
- Having gratitude
- Cultivating love, faith, and devotion
- Developing consciousness that we all need each other (unity)
- Viewing obstacles as opportunities to make changes
- Believing in abundance
- Taking risks in the name of growth and evolution
- Above all, practicing living in the present at all moments

The Detox Path

Why is detoxification necessary in today's world? Detoxification of body, mind, and soul is necessary in life for us to be able to more fully feel the true essence of the self and to prevent further physical and mental illness and disturbances. Detoxification of body, mind, and spirit is certainly a solution to live life in complete health, harmony, and prosperity.

The detoxification of the body-mind realm is a natural process that occurs to maintain the balance and strength in the body or mind. Unfortunately, in the world today, due to excess pollution, variations of food, deep stress, and the change of era, the human being is in need of finding tools to help activate the process of detoxification. The aim of the practice of yoga is to promote the path of detoxification and purification of the body, mind, and spirit; and it is probably one of the best alternatives in that it offers growth in peace and love as well as in health.

Presented here is a partial idea of how toxins come into our bodies and what we can do to prevent these toxins from staying and developing illness and disease. Considering the digestive system, the internal organs are probably the highest responsibility for the whole idea of detoxification. The food we eat, the liquids we drink, and the air we breathe need to be absorbed and transformed into nutrients for the body to work efficiently.

The process of digestion starts with the chewing of food in the mouth and finishes with the elimination of waste through the anus. Along this path there is a long way to run, with the participation of different organs involved.

The best way to nourish the body is with clean, organic fruits and vegetables, and with the assimilation of proteins derived from tofu and whole and clean organic cereals. As we learned in our sattvic diet lesson, we already know that the fewer toxins we accumulate in the organism, the better health we will have.

The way we cause stress in the digestive track is by overeating, eating food with poor fiber, eating the bulk of processed and refined foods and sugars, not getting enough water, and abusing drugs, alcohol, and medicines. When we practice yoga, an inside massage is provided, and the blood is stimulated to penetrate in every single area of the body to help purify the depth of each cell. It isn't enough to change the diet; we also need to vigorously exercise the body frequently.

The intestinal track is responsible for the digestion of food. It gets stressed because of the poisons that stay in the intestines and cannot be eliminated easily. This also negatively affects the circulation of blood and the lymphatic system.

The liver, the largest organs of the digestive system, evaluates every single substance that goes into the rest of the body. The main mission of the liver is to convert food into nutrition and remove toxins. It holds vitamins, breaks down sugars and hormones, and removes allergens, toxins, and funguses from the blood. It also helps the function of the gallbladder, where bile is generated, and is responsible for carrying away waste and breaking down fats in the digestion.

When the liver is sluggish and doesn't filter properly, signs of fatigue, depression, anger, digestion problems, cancer, diabetes, and difficulty in losing or gaining weight can manifest in the individual.

The liver needs to find detoxification through the journey so it can always function well.

The kidneys receive toxins from the liver, remove waste products, maintain the level of water, release hormones, and regulate blood pressure.

Not enough water, too much alcohol, additional and recreational drugs, mercury, aluminum, and other toxic metals in the body are responsible for a slow function of the kidneys.

The skin (the dermal system) is the largest organ for the elimination processes. It takes in and releases oxygen; when there is a lack of minerals and vitamins, the dermal system cannot work properly. Signs of acne, eczema, skin cancer, and so forth occur. Different complaints of the skin are the cause of a poor and general weak system. Many toxins enter into the body through care products such as creams, soaps, shampoos, toothpaste, ointments, and so forth.

These products can carry a great and enormous quantity of additives, colorants, animal components, and so forth. It is recommended to use care products and toothpaste with natural components.

In feminine pads and tampons, we find dioxins and chemical components that can generate bleeding and cause chemical burns inside the vagina. Stay away from conventional pads and tampons, and use unbleached organic qualities and brands.

Antiperspirants and deodorants fail to allow the release of toxins. Underneath the arm there are thousands of little glands that need to expel toxins. If the cycle of detoxification in this area doesn't happen properly, cancer and deviations of it can occur. Start using natural deodorants and avoid synthetic antiperspirants from now on.

As we have already learned, the body needs water, protein, carbohydrates, fat, vitamins, minerals, and enzymes to stay healthy. Enzymes are very important in the development of great health and are found in raw foods. The role of enzymes is to regenerate, break down, and digest foods, as well as deliver nutrients to the blood. Cooking food above 180 degrees destroys the enzymes. It is recommended that we eat raw food at least twice a day with organic salads, fruits, and raw vegetables. No healing can occur without enzymes.

The human body is made of 60 percent water; having enough water in the body helps to improve digestion and eliminate waste. The body needs to keep hydrated. Studies and statistics show that more than 85 percent of illnesses develop because of dryness in the system.

Air pollution affects everyone on the planet. Both outdoor and indoor pollution exists. When staying indoors, use natural fibers, cook with stainless cookware, reduce the use of electromagnetic fields, and avoid smoking or being in ambient of smoke, alcohol, and recreational drugs.

There is the moral and ethical part of not eating dead animals, but also there is the physical part. Chemicals, antibiotics hormones, additives, and so forth introduced into animals strongly impact the health of our bodies. We need to know that when we eat animal products we are also ingesting all kinds of additional poisons that increase the process of toxicity.

That's not to mention the state of terror animals go through before they are killed in slaughterhouses; this state releases adrenaline into the bloodstream. Human beings become exposed to the physical results of this fear and panic. Fish can have accumulations of aluminum, mercury, bacteria, and fungus due to pollution in the oceans.

Mind-Body Relationship with Detoxification

From the physical realm, we move into the emotional experience, where we find faith, hope, and, desire. We can keep our minds open to growth.

Yoga recognizes that there is no separation between the body parts, so our memories have influence over the function of the cells.

Love brings good vibrations while hate stands for bad vibration. When feelings of hate, jealousy, judgment, negativity, disappointment, and dissatisfaction appear and are not processed or eliminated, misalignments such as anxiety, stress, and fear will impact the system, leaving the body open to disease, anxiety, confusion, and depression.

We can have the best diet, yoga practice, and walks in nature; but if we aren't willing to open the experience to love and be willing to be open to change, difficulties will keep appearing in our path. And with that I am coming to the point: it isn't so important what you eat or what you think but who is eating you or who is thinking for you ... This is what really determines the state of your health. We all must look for spiritual freedom or salvation.

Change of mood invites responsibility. As we know in this life, everything happens intentionally for a spiritual purpose.

Bad moments will come, and challenges will appear. People we love will go. Everything comes to us because, in one way or another, we have been calling it, waiting for it; we invite our problems and disease. And I know this doesn't sound too fair or good, but we cannot remember our past times and lives, and karma can appear at any moment.

God always exists in good and bad moments. He is always present to embrace you, hold you, and protect you; no matter what, there is karma to clean and purify. Karma appears as a teacher to show where there is disconnection from truth, from light, and from God.

You have the power of choice to live your life as you like so you can live as a victim, blame, and complain. Or you can live with gratitude and happiness; it is your choice.

We face a transformational time of change. The divine program has entered into the baptism of fire. That means every day the power of fire increases in earth, creating general disasters, incurables disease, economical problems, depression, and inconvenient states of health. Ignorance of this event is the root of inn acceptance and misunderstands of humankind. For more information, log in to http://www.sukyomahikari.org and receive divine light.

In our spiritual practice, we chant, meditate, and receive divine light. We are open to the possible transformation, and we want this program to reinforce and grow every day more and more. Look for opportunities to expose the soul to the light, knowing that all you do is remember all you already know and return to your own and true origin.

Keep the practice of yoga active and pure so you can approach with independence and freedom the bright inner state of consciousness to facilitate the truth state of your mind. Then the connection between you and God's will is on during all times.

Anatomy of Movement: Physical

The anatomy of movement of the human body involves three systems of movement: The bones of the skeleton are linked with the joints and moved by the action of the muscles, opening the concept that the body moves through the kinetic chain.

The body can be moved in many different directions, and often more than one joint is involved. There are three different planes of movement we describe in relation to standard anatomical position, in which the body stays with feet parallel, arms hanging by the sides, palms and face directed forward.

Planes of Movement

The sagittal plane divides the body between right and left halves, and achieves movement through flexion and extension.

- Flexion—this takes part of the body forward from the anatomical position of flexion of the hip, shoulders, knee, neck, and so forth.
- Extension—this takes part of the body backward from anatomical position through extension of the neck, shoulders, hips, and so forth.
- Asana—Uttanasana, Utkatasana, Adho Mukha Svanasana

The frontal plane divides the body into anterior and posteriors parts, front and back. The movements are seen from the front.

- Adduction—this takes part of the body toward the center line; adduction of the hip is the crossing of the leg toward the medial line.
- Abduction—this takes part of the body away from the middle line; abduction of the shoulder is raising the arm.
- Lateral flexion—this is from the side of the trunk, bending to one side.
- Asana—Uttitha Trikonasana, Viradhadrasana II, and Ardha Chandrasana

The transverse plane: divides the body into superior and inferior—upper and lower parts.

- Lateral rotation—movement that occurs when part of the body rotates outward. Lateral rotation of the hip is opening the foot and rotating the hip.
- Medial rotation movement occurs when part of the body rotates inward. This is the medial rotation of the shoulder part, moved internally.
- Parivrtta Trikonasana, Ardha Matsyendrasana, Parivrtta Utkatasana

The Skeleton

The skeleton is a mobile framework of bones; it provides rigid support for the body and bones, serving as levers for the action of the muscles.

There are three basic shapes of bones: long bones (femur), short bones (ankle), and flat bones (scapula). The tissue of the bones is composed of calcium and salts that bring rigidity and elasticity.

Anatomy of the Knee

The knee is one of the most used joints in the body. Probably it is the most flexible, mobile, and abused of joints, so that leads it to be one of the most injured parts of the body. The femur (thighbone), patella (kneecap), and tibia (shinbone) are the three bones attached to the knee.

The knee lies halfway between the hip and the ankle; it is involved in all the actions of the legs; the stabilization and alignment of the knee come from ligaments and tendons attached to the bones. The anterior and posterior ligaments cross one another in the center of the knee. The ligaments function together to limit rotation and separately to prevent the tibia from moving forward—ACL—and the femur from moving backward—PCL. On the sides of the knee is another set of stabilizing ligaments called collateral ligaments; they provide stabilization, preventing the knee from moving side to side when someone does sharp and cutting moves.

The patella is a sesamoid bone (bone with tendon) that lies in the quadriceps, changes the angle, serves to protect the tendon from wearing out, and acts as a shock absorber. An articular cartilage protects the knee joint, covering the ends of the tibia and femur.

The menisci are thin pads of strong, fibrous tissues that are mobile and aid to spread synovial fluid during the knee movements. The menisci also act as shock absorbers, cushioning the join of impact and providing knee stability.

Muscles of the Knee

- Knee flexors (front) and quadriceps (rectus femoris, vastus lateralis, vastus medialis, and vastus intermedius)
- Knee extensors (back), hamstrings (semimembranosus, semitendinosus, and biceps femurus), gastrocnemius, and soleus
- Medial and lateral rotators—on sides and intermediate muscles

Variation of Knee's Positions

- Knees into center line with feet apart (knock–knee/valgus)
- Knees away from center line with feet together (bowlegged/valgus)
- Hyperextension
- Patella facing in
- Patella facing out

Anatomy of the Foot and Ankle (Foundation)

The feet and ankles bear the weight of the body and are responsible for all the movements that allow us to walk, run, dance, and so forth. This area of the body contains numerous bones and joint structures that bring a combination of flexibility and strength. It is important to take care of the area and wear comfortable shoes that will positively affect the health of the foot and ankle.

The ankle joint connects the tibia with the talus. The joint is responsible for extension and flexion.

Alignment of the Foot

When standing barefoot, the foot should toe out slightly so the longitudinal arch can be visible and create a half-moon shape; the toes should be relaxed and extend forward in line with the foot. As you walk, the feet should move in parallel with the weight transferred from the lateral border of the heel to the ball of the foot.

Reflexology Points of the Foot

- Toes: heart, lungs, and related organs of the face (nose, eyes, and ears)
- Arches: digestive organs (stomach, liver, pancreas, gallbladder, and intestines)
- Heels: related to kidneys and sexual organs

Elbow

The elbow relates to the movements of our hands. The bones—ulna, radius, and humerus—articulate in the elbow. The elbow is designed to provide maximum stability as we use the forearms and hands. Like the knee, the elbow depends on ligaments to stabilize and support it. The elbow is a fragile bone structure; the ligaments connect the humerus to the ulna; also, several important tendons aid elbow movement. The biceps tendon attaches the bicep muscle during the elbow flexion; the antagonist or counteraction is the triceps. It allows the elbow to straighten with force, for example, in Chaturanga Dandasana. Common problems with the elbow and wrist involve nerves and certainly can affect the shoulders and create tendonitis or carpal tunnel disorder.

Wrist

Wrists and hands are capable of performing endless movements of any complexity. The radius and ulna also meet at the hands to form the wrists; the hand is made of many small bones, including carpal, metacarpal, and phalanges. The hand is so complex that it reminds us of the foot.

The upper extremities are capable of a great variety of movement. A good alignment of the shoulders is essential following the position of the rib cage.

Hand and wrist alignment is essential to prevent nerve disorders. Hands and feet are the parts of the body that ground us to the earth in the practice of yoga; they need to be in good alignment to prevent injuries, and we find the maximum strength and movement through them.

Remember that the body learns movement by doing it—good patterns develop with time and quality of movement.

Glossary: Physical Anatomy

- Distal: structure farther from the midpoint
- Proximal: structure closer to the midpoint
- Posterior: back of the body
- Anterior: front of the body
- Supine: lying on the back, facing up
- Pronation: lying on the front, facing down
- Joints: articulations of bones
- Ligaments: tissue that connects bone to bone
- Tendon: tissue that connects bone with muscle
- Sciatic nerve: largest nerve of lumbosacral muscles
- Sacrum: the sacred bone, the lowermost major segment of the spine; five pairs of spinal nerves exit in the sacrum.
- Perineum: a diamond–shaped region that hammocks the bottom of the pelvic basin
- Agonist: muscles or group of muscles that creates movement
- Antagonist: a muscle that opposes the function of another on the opposite side of the bone by restraining movement of the joint
- Range of motion: number of degrees that a joint allows one of its segments to move

Shapes of the Spine

The art of knowing how to move the body corrects posture, revitalizes physical mobility, invigorates the mind, and elevates the spirit. The body knows nothing of muscles; the body knows only movement. The need to educate the muscles in appropriate movement pervades all aspects in our lives. The way we move is reflected in our posture and gestures. Our movements, in essence, tell the story of our lives, holding the blueprints of our bodies, minds, and spirits. That is why it's important not only how we move but also what we say and what thoughts come to our minds and contribute to patterns of mental habit.

During movement on the mat, the body makes constant changes to preserve equilibrium, coordinating hundreds of muscles that work simultaneously. Significantly, muscle imbalances always appear in two major areas of the body: the pelvic complex and the shoulder complex. These lead to faulty movement patterns that reverberate through the entire body.

Because yoga and Pilates put the body in motion, promote circulation, and teach proper movement and control, they can counter the strains of our daily habituated postures and enhance overall muscular balance.

Good health depends on good posture, full breathing, good nutritional balance, and centered thoughts and feelings. The body's posture is a mirror that reflects the internal self to the outside world with ideas, attitudes, and feelings. In our posture we exhibit the way we are: our self–confidence, self–esteem, and self-realization.

Good posture can be described as the following: heels together, the weight distributed between two feet, legs together in the center line, abdominals lifting in and up, decompressing the spine, sternum forward and up, shoulders relaxed and down, and the rib cage above the back of the hips, with ears and eyes level.

Poor posture is often a combination of different factors and may block the circuits of energy through the spine and the channels of life–force. Some factors that favor bad posture in the human being are the following: hereditary influences, gravitational force, hours of sitting and remaining static (this starts in school), injuries, muscle imbalances, insufficient exercises, lack of awareness, adopting bad postures over the desk, or carrying too much weight on the shoulders (backpacks or extra-full handbags).

Bad habits lead the body to bad posture, and then we can suffer from strained back muscles, which lead to poor circulation to the head and provoke dizziness, chronic fatigue, migraines, and chronic lower back pain. Compression of the chest with a rounded upper back can affect breathing. And so, with shallow breathing and poor oxygen supply, internal organs can be affected; also digestive problems, among many others conditions, can occur.

Different patterns and deviations of poor posture can certainly affect alignment of movement and can then affect the kinetic chain. The major postural deviations of the spine presented in the general population are the following:

- Lordosis posture (hollow back syndrome): exaggerated anterior curvature of the lumbar spine often results in a protruding abdomen and buttocks. Normally it is associated with lower back pain, weak gluteal muscles, anterior pelvic tilt, tight lower back, weak abdominal muscles, weak thoracic extensors, and weak and tight hip flexors. It is appropriate to work with emphasis in the abdominal muscles to strengthen the weak muscles and decompress the spine.
- Kyphosis posture: kyphosis can occur either in the lumbar or in the thoracic spine region. When present in the lumbar spine, it creates a flat back; when present in the upper back, it leads to a rounded spine. It compromises the ability to absorb shock, which in the long term deteriorates health and speeds the breakdown of the vertebral disks.
- Kyphosis lumbar posture: pelvis forward, weak spinal erectors, tight spinal flexors, tight upper abdominals, and tight hamstrings
- Kyphosis thoracic posture: tight anterior shoulder girdle, weak upper back, weak cervical muscles, and tight upper abdominals
- Many movements we do in yoga and Pilates strengthen the upper body and emphasize the full breath so kyphosis can be reduced; decompressing the spine and building abdominal strength, teaching how to initiate movement from the center.

Lordotic/kyphotic combination posture: exaggerated lordotic lumbar curve, a rounded thoracic curve with a forward thrust of neck and head, weak abdominals, weak gluteal. This problem includes hyperextended knee joints, tight chest muscles, weak upper back muscles, weak cervical muscles, and an anterior pelvic tilt.

Focusing on strengthening the abdominal muscles will help to address the hollow of the lumbar spine and to align and reinforce the upper body. Also, it will be helpful to stretch the anterior upper torso with standing positions.

Swayback posture: often confused with lordosis, swayback is different. Normally the pelvis is in the anterior tilt position and held forward from the center line; it is also known as "lazy posture." With poor muscle action, the muscles don't provide support; instead the person yields to gravity, resulting in the pelvis being forward, extension of hips, and extension of the lumbar spine forward. With the shoulders and head forward, the posture arrives from a slouched posture, with fatigue, muscle weakness, and poor exercise designs. For these individuals, it is good to emphasize reeducating them, waking up the upper muscles, and teaching proper movement from the core.

Scoliosis: a curvature of the spine; scoliosis affects the muscles and ligaments of the spinal column. Scoliosis can cause neurological, hormonal, and digestive symptoms and vary on an individual basis; it can intervene in limitation of rotation.

Vertebras and the Spine

The spinal column is made up of twenty-six vertebrae—seven cervical, twelve thoracic, and five lumbar, the sacrum, and the coccyx. All the vertebrae are connected and aligned by a system of joints, ligaments, and muscles that provide movement and stability. Between each vertebra lie the vertebrae disks, which are composed of cartilage and fibrous tissue rotation. In the middle of the vertebrae disks there is a gelatin–like substance. Herniation occurs when the disks tear and the gelatin bulges; in extreme cases the bulging becomes painful when the gel presses against the spinal nerves.

The natural curves of the spine are vitally important. They allow the spine to act as a shock absorber during activities such as walking, running, jumping, doing yoga, performing Pilates, and so forth.

Movements of the spine include the following:

Flexion—Uttanasana
Lateral flexion—Trikonasana
Extension—Bhujangasana
Hyperextension—Urdhva Dhanurasana
Rotation on same side—Ardha Chandrasana
Rotation on other side—Parivrtta Trikonasana

In movements of body-mind-spirit modalities, the concept is to lengthen the spine and create space between vertebrae, knowing that the three segments of the spine (lumbar, thoracic, and cervical) are able to extend, lengthen, and reinforce with each movement and breath.

The muscles of the spine can be superficial or deep:

- Superficial muscles are in control of the limbs and the respiratory system.
- Deep muscles act to maintain postural control and move the vertebral column.

The anterior muscles of the spine are the abdominal muscles, which stabilize and protect the column, supporting internal organs and providing grace and control to the movement. They link the pelvis with the rib cage. There are four major muscles:

- Rectus abdominis
- External oblique
- Internal oblique
- Transversus abdominis

These muscles don't attach to bones; they attach to fascia (sheets of connective tissue that support and give form to organs and muscles through the body).

The Pelvis

It is said that life begins in the pelvis. The pelvis is the center of stability and originator of life and motion. The pelvis is the bridge between the torso and the lower limbs. Any large movement we do involves the shift of the pelvis. Misalignments of the pelvis affect the angle of the hips, the lumbar spine, and the body in general.

Structure of the pelvis: pelvis shape differs from individual to individual. Women tend to have a broader, larger pelvic cavity, while men have a thicker, heavier, and narrower structure.

The pelvis is formed by three very important coxal bones or hip bones, which fuse together after infancy: ilium, ischium, and pubis.

- The ilium is the wing–shaped structure and the larger component; it holds the acetabulum (hip socket) from where the head of the femur and the pelvis articulate.
- The ischium forms the seat bones.
- The pubis is the lower anterior and inferior bone of the pelvis that contributes to the formation of the pubic symphysis.

Alignment of the pelvis prevents injury, is essential to strengthen the lumbar spine, and promotes healthy movement patterns. Important pelvic elements are the following:

- ASIS: pelvis forward
- PSIS: pelvis back
- Sacrum: larger portion of the spine that intersects the pelvis
- The iliac crest: the top edge of the ilium; it can be felt when placing hands on hips.

Muscles of the pelvic region: twenty-nine muscles cross the pelvis region and affect the function of the area formed by spinal extensors, abdominals, quadratus lumborum, and iliopsoas. These muscles play a great role in the spinal movement and are responsible for health in the spine.

The Pelvic Floor Musculature (in Yoga: Mula Bhanda)

The pelvic floor is like the hammock that cradles the abdominal organs. The muscles work to support and elevate the organs of the pelvic cavity, including the reproductive organs and bladder. It is very important to keep these muscles strong to prevent injuries in the lower back.

The Hips

The large and mobile ball and socket joint of the hip is formed from the articulation of the acetabulum and the head of the femur. Because the femur is a long bone that extends to the knee joint, the movement of the pelvis affects the lower kinetic chain, affecting the way we walk and run.

The Breath

It is said that the first act of life is to breathe, and so it is also the last.

The flow of breath affects physical and mental stress, and can interfere in changes through the day. The average adult breathes twenty-six thousand times a day. The breath performed correctly offers rejuvenation and invigorates the mind; however, if breathing is poor and incorrect, restriction of the respiratory system will happen.

The ways to take air in and out are simply by the mouth or the nose. To approach optimal health, breathe well, exercise well, and eat correctly.

Anatomy of the Shoulders and Cervical Spine

In a complex sense, we can say that yoga and Pilates help to restore the natural function of the body by exercising the muscles to improve their efficiency and range of movement. This tends to be a benefit for the human form, improving the appearance and proportion of the body. As the body and movement fuse together, they flow together, creating different shapes in the space. As a result and with time and persistence, we create a strong center with long musculature. The neuromuscular and skeletal system of the body gets in a revolution state as it aligns one body part with another.

In two major areas of the body, the pelvic complex and the shoulder complex, we find the most areas of imbalances, and these lead to faulty movement patterns. Reinforcing and aligning these two major areas will lead to the benefit of the exercise and help to maintain the body in optimal heath and posture.

The Shoulder Complex

The structure of the shoulder provides a very large motion in the upper body; the shoulder is one of the most mobile joints of the body. The shoulder complex is a structure made up of three joints: the glenohumeral joint, the acromioclavicular joint, and the sternoclavicular joint. The primary joint of the shoulder is the glenohumeral; the framework of this joint is made up of two scapulae and two clavicles.

The clavicles attach the sternum in the center, and they connect the arms with the thorax. It's important to know that the shoulder complex doesn't attach to the spine; the internal organs of the heart and lungs are protected by the shoulder complex. In addition, the nonattachment of the shoulder complex to the spine helps to free the arms for powerful movement over a wide range of motion without causing pressure on internal organs.

The scapulae form the two wider and triangular bones that glide over the back of the rib cage. They float over the posterior rib cage, suspended by a network of muscles and ligaments. The scapula reaches toward the front and side of the body.

Movements of the shoulder complex include the following:

- Flexion: arms lift forward in a sagittal plane.
- Extension: arms lift back in a sagittal plane.
- Abduction: arms lift away from midline in a frontal plane.
- Adduction: arms go back to the body in a frontal plane.

- External rotation: humerus rotates forward in a transverse plane.
- Internal rotation: humerus rotates inward to the transverse plane (Plank).

Almost every bone in the trunk is in contact with some portion of the shoulder complex, extending to all directions: upward to the head, around the rib cage, from spine to sternum, and through the entire length of the back. The muscles of the shoulder complex can be divided into three groups:

Group 1: from scapula to humerus, we find the rotator group of muscles; those are supraspinatus, infraspinatus, teres minor, and subscapularis.

Group 2: from torso to scapula, these muscles work hard to stabilize the scapula, hold it in place against the thorax, and maintain the correct posture of the head, upper body, and spine.

Group 3: from torso to humerus includes large and flat muscles that rise from the torso and pass through the upper arm, providing strength and range of motion; pectorals major, deltoids, latissimus dorsi, and serratus anterior.

Movements of the Scapula

Abduction/protraction: moves the scapula forward and apart from one another

Adduction: moves the scapula toward the spine; moves them toward one another

Elevations: moves the scapula toward the head

Depression: moves the scapula toward the pelvis

Inward rotation: draws the outer tip of the scapula upward medially

If there is an imbalance in the alignment of the spine, the shoulder complex will be modified. Working appropriately with alignment of the pelvis and the spine will benefit the posture of the shoulders. The movement of the arms should adjust the shoulders. The arm movements affect the thoracic spine and rib cage. They are all connected.

The Cervical Spine

The head is a heavy load sitting atop the spinal column; the skull makes contact with the first vertebra (atlas) via small, shallow projections called the occipital condyles, found in the base of the skull. The atlas rests on the axis (second vertebra), which allows the rotation of the skull. Thanks to this vertebra, the head can be carried easily and provide a great range of motion.

Any deviation of the head produces a huge impact on the entire body because it produces a modification of the center of gravity. When the head is off center, the cervical spine's curve is disturbed, and the sense of orientation can be modified.

The organs of the inner ear convey information with the eye muscles, allowing the eyes to adapt to new levels of vision. Over time the eyes and body will adapt to a faulty posture, and what is wrong habitually feels right and normal.

Appropriate exercise for the muscles of the neck and cervical spine will prevent any modification from the right alignment of this area. Because the upper cervical spine is linked to the sensory organs, problems that include injuries, respiratory problems, and chronic joint pain can occur easily.

The Muscles of the Spine

Head and neck muscles are very strong, allowing balance and moving the heavy skull and brain. A series of wires from the skull to the ribs, sternum, scapulae, and clavicles provide strength on all sides. Trapezius, sternocleidomastoid, and prevertebral muscles work together to control the position of the head.

Because of poor postural position or bad habits (working too many hours at a desk, for example), those muscles can become weak, producing little control over the orientation and placement of the head when lifting it in a supine position. It is important to work with students to strengthen the muscles of the neck in the correct alignments to improve posture.

People are creatures of habit. Faulty and habitual posture and movement, a sedentary lifestyle, insufficient movement, and poor training can skew movement patterns. Common problems seen in the upper areas of the body relate to lower areas. When a movement cannot be achieved by a muscle or a series of them, the body will adapt, using a trick muscle easily. In other words, it is easy for the body to trick movements with inappropriate muscles. The natural state for the body is to have the head aligned over the pelvis. To find good posture, look for ideal alignment of head, neck, and torso with pelvis, knees, ankle, and foot position. The good function of the nervous system retrains movements. When one is learning new asana or exercises, because the movement is unfamiliar, muscles are often tight, and the body struggles. This is the reason to keep practicing familiar exercises and introducing the patterns of new exercises, improving posture, developing strength, and obtaining progress in body, mind, and spirit.

The strength and power of the Pilates method is always determined by directions, and it quotes what the creator Joseph Pilates (1880–1967) taught in the world.

Be aware.
Achieve balance.
Breathe correctly.
Concentrate deeply.
Center yourself.
Gain control.
Become efficient.
Create flow.
Become precise.
Seek harmony.

Chapter 4

Warm-Up

Center
Neck Roll
Lateral Stretching
Center Arms Side to Namaste
Cat-Cow in Siddhasana
Chakravakasana-Balasana

Warm-up typically includes some preliminary stretching of the neck, shoulders, arms, back, lateral core muscles, legs, and so forth. This is usually done in a more or less controlled form led by the instructor and may include controlled breathing.

Warm-up teaches the teacher the condition of the student.

Warm-up is completely optional and depends on the teacher. However, between opening, breathing control, and warm-up in a vinyasa format, we wouldn't exceed ten minutes.

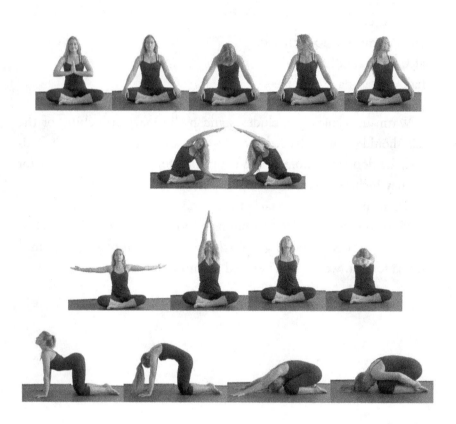

Chapter 5

Surya Namaskar A and B

Surya Namaskar A
1. Tadasana or Samasthiti
2. Urdhva Hasta Sirsasana
3. Uttanasana
4. Ardha Uttanasana
5. Chaturanga Dandasana
6. Urdhva Mukha Svanasana
7. Adho Mukha Svanasana

Ardha Uttanasana
Uttanasana
Urdhva Hasta Sirsasana
Tadasana or Samasthiti

Surya Namaskar B

Tadasana or Samasthiti
8. Utkatasana
Uttanasana
Ardha Uttanasana
Chaturanga Dandasana
Urdhva Mukha Svanasana
Adho Mukha Svanasana
Virabhadrasana I (Right)
Chaturanga Dandasana
Urdhva Mukha Svanasana
Adho Mukha Svanasana
9. Virabhadrasana I (Left)

Chaturanga Dandasana

Marta Berry

Urdhva Mukha Svanasana
Adho Mukha Svanasana
Ardha Uttanasana
Uttanasana
Utkatasana
Tadasana or Samasthiti

Tadasana or Samasthiti—Mountain Pose

Skill: Beginner
Breath: Three
Drishti: Forward
Goal: To Correct Posture and Bring Awareness of the Body
Category: Standing Position

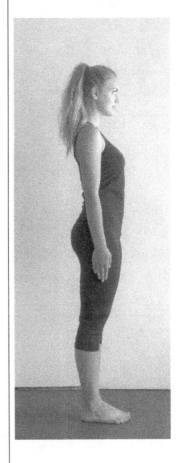

Technique
Stand up with feet and legs together. Find the internal good posture. Maintain the backs of the shoulders on top of the backs of the hips. Put hands on the hips

Modification
Keep the feet width distance apart.

Cues—Teaching Tips
Keep the back straight, lift the kneecaps up, and maintain the shoulders down.

Energetic Benefits
It relaxes the body, brings stability and freedom of movement, and refreshes the circulation.

Physical Benefits
It lengthens the body, brings awareness, and corrects posture.

Notes:

Urdhva Hasta Sirsasana—Arms Up

Skill: Beginner
Breath: Inhale—1
Drishti: Thumbs
Goal: To Lengthen the Spine and the Body
Category: Standing Position

Technique
From Tadasana, lift the arms up, keep your hands together, and gaze at the thumbs.

Modification
Keep feet and hands width distance apart.

Cues—Teaching Tips
Keep the back straight, lift the kneecaps up, and maintain the shoulders down.

Energetic Benefits
It brings confidence, enhances self–esteem, and delivers peace and tranquility.

Physical Benefits
It lengthens the body, favors circulation toward the heart, and creates space between the neck and shoulders.

Notes:

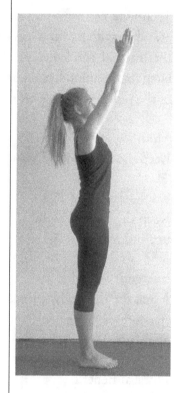

Uttanasana—Forward Fold

Skill: Beginner

Breath: Exhale—1

Drishti: Knees

Goal: To Invert the Position of the Body, Soothing the Nervous System

Category: Standing Position, Forward Fold

Technique
From Urdhva Hasta Sirsasana, hinge from the hips and go forward all the way down. The hands rest beside the feet, and the head faces the floor.

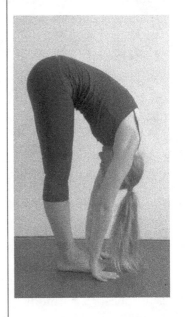

Modification
Keep the feet width distance apart, bend the knees, and use a block.

Cues—Teaching Tips
Keep the back straight and lift the kneecaps. Keep the sitting bones above the heels.

Energetic Benefits
It alleviates anxiety and depression, and it allows one to be open for gratitude and changes.

Physical Benefits
It tones the internal organs, relieves stomach ailments, and soothes the nervous system.

Notes:

Ardha Uttanasana—Half Forward Fold

Skill: Beginner
Breath: Inhale—1
Drishti: Forward
Goal: To Elongate the Spine and Prepare for Chaturanga Dandasana
Category: Standing Position

Technique
From Uttanasana, lengthen the back so it is parallel to the floor.

Modification
Keep the feet width distance apart, bend the knees, and place hands on thighs or block.

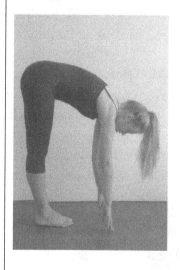

Cues—Teaching Tips
Keep the back straight, lift the kneecaps, and keep the shoulders away from the neck.

Energetic Benefits
It empowers energy, pleasure, and joy. It establishes self-harmony.

Physical Benefits
It elongates back muscles, teaches one to keep shoulder blades in place, and brings awareness of a flat back.

Notes:

Chaturanga Dandasana—Plank Pose

Skill: Beginner
Breath: Exhale—1
Drishti: Forward
Goal: To Manage the Weight of the Body
Category: Abdominal Work, Shoulder Opener

Technique
From Ardha Uttanasana, jump to Chaturanga Dandasana and bend the elbows.

Modification
With knees on the floor, lie down completely on the floor.

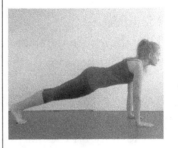

Cues—Teaching Tips
Keep the elbows tucked into the body. Keep the backs of the legs and buttocks strong. Make sure heels reach back and stay off the floor.

Energetic Benefits
It helps to move forward, learning from the best experiences of the past.

Physical Benefits
It strengthens the upper body, wrists, arms, and abdominal muscles. It aligns the body and increases power and mobility.

Notes:

Urdhva Mukha Svanasana—Upward Dog

Skill: Beginner
Breath: Inhale—1
Drishti: Forward, Upward
Goal: To Lengthen the Back and Prepare for Back Bends
Category: Back Bend

Technique
From Chaturanga Dandasana, flatten the feet and change the position of the body. Lower the hips, pressing them forward and off the floor. Keep your arms straight and shoulders back.

Modification
Keep the legs on the floor. Extend the back like in Bhujangasana (with elbows bended).

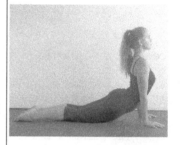

Cues—Teaching Tips
It teaches one how to control the weight of the body off the mat, with strength in the back. Push with the tips of the feet and hands, and open the shoulders. The chest is off the floor.

Energetic Benefits
It vitalizes and refreshes, combats indecision, and promotes general health, courage, and hope.

Physical Benefits
It rejuvenates the spine, brings elasticity to the lungs, and improves sciatica, lumbago, and even slipped disk.

Notes:

Adho Mukha Svanasana—Down Dog

Skill: Beginner
Breath: Five
Drishti: Navel
Goal: To Stretch the Body in Opposition
Category: Standing Position

Technique
From Urdhva Mukha Svanasana, lift the hips and shape the body in a V posture. Spread fingers wide apart and place feet hip-width distance apart. Lift hips to the sky and pull back legs strongly.

Modification
Bend the knees and shorten the stand with hands on blocks.

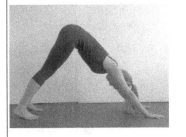

Cues—Teaching Tips
Lift the hips, anchor the heels down, and keep the shoulders wide and in place.

Energetic Benefits
Establish self-confidence, self-honor, and equilibrium in thought.

Physical Benefits
It relieves stiffness from shoulders, lengthens the spine, reduces fatigue, lengthens the body, and brings awareness of posture.

Notes:

Utkatasana—Chair Pose

Skill: Beginner
Breath: Inhale—1
Drishti: Thumbs
Goal: To Lengthen the Spine
Category: Standing Position

Technique
From Tadasana, bend the knees and drop
the hips toward the floor, lift the back,
and raise the arms above the head. Touch
the palms and look at the thumbs.

Modification
Keep the feet hip-width distance apart,
bend the knees less, and keep hands apart.

Cues—Teaching Tips
Keep the back straight, squeeze the knees
and hips together, and breathe deeply.

Energetic Benefits
It establishes total connection between
body and mind, relaxes actions, and
creates compassion for others.

Physical Benefits
It develops leg muscles evenly, fully
expands the chest, and massages the heart
and internal organs.

Notes:

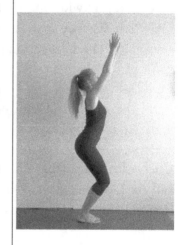

Virabhadrasana I—Warrior I

Skill: Beginner
Breath: Inhale—1
Drishti: Thumbs
Goal: To Find Victory over Actions and Empower the Will
Category: Standing Position

Technique
Standing with feet apart (three to four feet), place the front foot out and the back foot in. Bend the front knee, keep the torso straight, raise the arms above the head, bring the hands together, and look up.

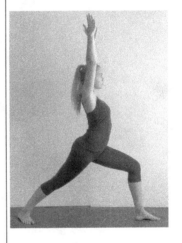

Modification
Shorten the stand. Bend the knees less, with arms straight forward or apart.

Cues—Teaching Tips
The back leg and foot provide the stability for the pose, which should be strong and grounded. The tailbone should come forward with the front knee bending deeply.

Energetic Benefits
It brings faith and power to the action, and it creates inner peace and acceptance of responsibilities.

Physical Benefits
It tones the ankles, knees, and hips. It relieves stiffness of the neck and shoulders. It fully expands the chest.

Notes:

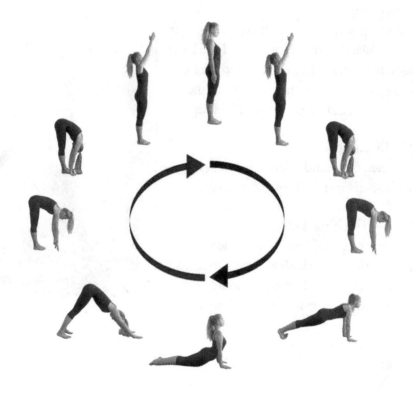

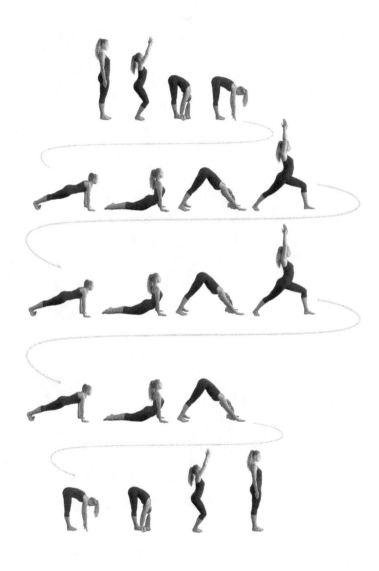

Chapter 6

Beginner Asana

Standing Positions
1. Padangusthasana
2. Padahastasana
3. Prasarita Padottanasana

Balance Positions
4. Vrksasana
5. Utthita Hasta Padangusthasana

Back Bends
6. Bhujangasana
7. Salabhasana

Sitting Positions
Forward Folds
8. Dandasana
9. Paschimottanasana

Hip Openers
10. Siddhasana
11. Baddha Konasana
12. Padmasana
13. Parvatasana

Twists
14. Marichyasana II
15. Marichyasana III

Abdominal Work

Pilates

    16. Single-Leg Stretch

    17. Double-Leg Stretch

    18. Single Straight-Leg Stretch

General Body Stretch

    19. Supta Baddha Konasana

    20. Supta Padangusthasana

    21. Anantasana

Inversions

    22. Sarvangasana

    23. Halasana

Padangusthasana—Big Toe

Skill: Beginner
Breath: Five
Drishti: Back
Goal: To Relax the Mind and Tone the Abdominal Organs
Category: Standing Position

Technique
From Tadasana, with feet apart and hands on hips, inhale and look up. Exhale, forward fold, and hold big toes. Inhale and look forward. Exhale with top of head down. To come out, inhale and look forward. Exhale with hands on hips. Inhale and come up.

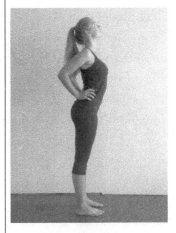

Modification
Bend the knees and grab the ankles.

Cues—Teaching Tips
Tuck the chin in and keep the legs strong. Lift shoulders.

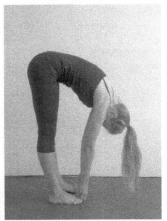

Energetic Benefits
It helps to control fearful emotions and brings a sense of peace and security. It assists one in making right decisions.

Physical Benefits
It tones the liver and spleen, soothes the nervous system, and favors circulation toward the heart.

Notes:

Padahastasana—Stretch Wrist Pose

Skill: Beginner
Breath: Five
Drishti: Back
Goal: To Strengthen the Wrist and Spine
Category: Standing Position

Technique
From Tadasana with feet apart, put hands on hips and inhale. Look up and exhale. Do a forward fold. Slide the palms under the soles of the feet, inhale, and look forward. Exhale with top of head down. To come out, inhale, look forward, and exhale with hands on hips. Inhale and come up.

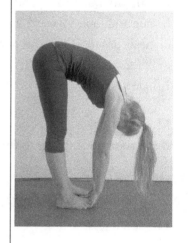

Modification
Bend the knees and grab the side of each foot.

Cues—Teaching Tips
Look back, relax the neck, and press the base of the wrist.

Energetic Benefits
It brings stability, frees the mind, and helps one to be focused.

Physical Benefits
It soothes the nervous system, activates internal organs, and maintains a calm mind.

Notes:

Prasarita Padottanasana—Stretch Pose

Skill: Beginner
Breath: Five
Drishti: Back
Goal: To Heal the Body and Stretch the Spine
Category: Standing Position

Technique
Legs should be four inches apart with arms straight at the sides. Inhale up and exhale down. Inhale and move forward. Exhale and move down.

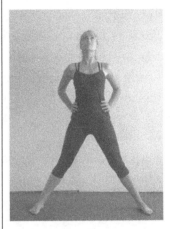

A. Put hands between legs.
B. Place hands on hips.
C. Interlace fingers behind and up.
D. Grab big toes.

Modification
Bend the knees. Don't interlace the fingers. Don't lower as much.

Cues—Teaching Tips
Relax the muscles of the middle spine. Lift the shoulders. Keep the legs strong. Tuck the chin in.

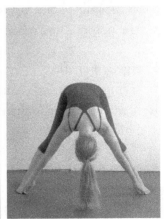

Energetic Benefits
It brings awareness of the present and helps one to set up new goals for the future.

Physical Benefits
It develops hamstrings and increases blood flow into the trunk and head. It reduce body weight.

Notes

Vrksasana—Tree Pose

Skill: Beginner
Breath: Five
Drishti: Forward
Goal: To Find Balance and Elongate the Spine
Category: Standing Position, Balance

Technique
From Tadasana bend one knee and place feet on the opposite inner thigh. Press firmly and grow taller. Extend arms over the head.

Modification
Keep the feet under the knee. Place it on a block and use the wall.

Cues—Teaching Tips
Push the pubic bone forward and look to a focal point. Grow taller.

Energetic Benefits
It brings security, confidence, and freedom of expression. It keeps one valiant and brave.

Physical Benefits
It tones the leg muscles, opens the hips and chest, and keeps one in balance.

Notes:

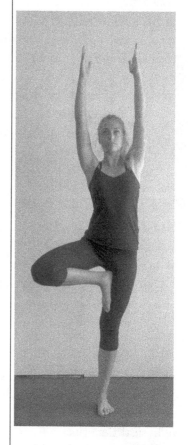

Utthita Hasta Padangusthasana— Stretch Big Toe Up

Skill: Beginner
Breath: Five
Drishti: Forward
Goal: To Reinforce the Muscle of the Legs
Category: Standing Position, Balance

Technique
From Tadasana bend one knee. Grab the big toe and extend the leg forward. Keep the opposite hand on the hip and balance the body.

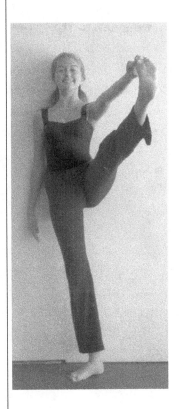

Modification
Keep the knee bent. Use a wall to find balance. Use a strap.

Cues—Teaching Tips
Open the chest, maintain strong leg muscles, and point the lifted foot.

Energetic Benefits
It releases trauma from the past and present. It comforts grief and self-pity. It brings efficiency and security.

Physical Benefits
It reinforces all the muscles in both legs. It stabilizes and completely calms the body.

Notes:

Bhujangasana—Snake Pose

Skill: Beginner
Breath: Three
Drishti: Forward
Goal: To Tone the Spinal Region
Category: Back Bend

Technique
Lying in a prone position, place hands under the shoulders with legs and feet together. Direct elbows toward the hips and inhale, lifting the chest. Exhale and lower.

Modification
Keep the legs and feet hip-width distance apart. Look down and use a blanket.

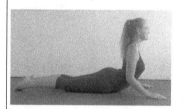

Cues—Teaching Tips
Press the pubic bone down and keep the elbows near the body. Let the head follow the spine.

Energetic Benefits
Let go of personal limitations. Enhance self-esteem and help with honesty.

Physical Benefits
It tones the spinal region and expands the chest, bringing slipped disks to their original position.

Notes:

Salabhasana —Locust Pose

Skill: Beginner
Breath: Five
Drishti: Forward
Goal: To Bring Elasticity in the Back
Category: Back Bend

Technique
Lying in a prone position, lift the following parts of the body off the floor: feet, legs, chest, arms, hands, neck, and head. Keep the hips on the floor.

Modification
Keep the feet width distance apart. Place a blanket under the belly.

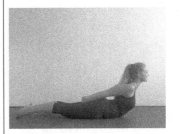

Cues—Teaching Tips
Keep the abdominal muscles engaged. Lift from the muscles of the upper back; keep the shoulder blades in their place.

Energetic Benefits
Easy the practice. It opens the heart to self-love and awakens new perspectives.

Physical Benefits
It aids digestion and relieves pain in the sacrum and lumbar area. It lengthens the body.

Notes:

Dandasana—Staff Pose

Skill: Beginner
Breath: Five
Drishti: Down
Goal: To Prepare the Body for Forward Folds, to Locate the Bandhas
Category: Sitting Position

Technique
Sit on the floor, legs straight and together in front. Flex the feet with arms straight, hands beside hips, and shins above the collarbone. Practice engaging the three bandhas (Maha Bandha).

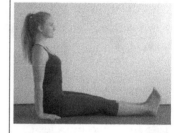

Modification
Place a blanket, bend the knees, and keep the legs separated.

Cues—Teaching Tips
Shape the form of the letter *L*. Place hands under shoulders and shoulder blades on place. Reach long with strong legs and feet in a flexed position.

Energetic Benefits
It enhances relationships, promotes pleasure in the actions, and improves vocal skills.

Physical Benefits
It releases tension of the stomach, helps gastric complaints, tones the kidneys, and removes waste around the waistline.

Notes:

Paschimottanasana—West Stretch Pose

Skill: Beginner
Breath: Five
Drishti: Down to Toes
Goal: To Rejuvenate the Spine
Category: Sitting Position, Forward Fold

Technique
From Dandasana, lift arms and fold them forward. Hold the feet or big toes.

Modification
Bend the knees. Using a strap, sit on a blanket and separate the legs.

Cues—Teaching Tips
Keep the back straight above the legs. Maintain the shoulders in their place and lengthen forward from the lower back.

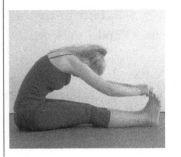

Energetic Benefits
It brings awareness and presence. It stimulates mind power and organizes power of choice.

Physical Benefits
It activates abdominal organs, tones the kidneys, and increases blood flow in pubic region.

Notes:

Siddhasana—Perfect Pose

Skill: Beginner
Breath: Five
Drishti: Forward
Goal: To Prepare for Meditation
Category: Sitting Position, Hip Opener

Technique
Sitting on the floor, cross one leg in front
of the other. Lengthen the spine and relax
the shoulders down.

Modification
Use a blanket to elevate the pelvis. Use
blocks under the knees.

Cues—Teaching Tips
Lower the knees and elevate the spine.
Keep the chin above the collarbone.
Extend the top of the head toward the
ceiling.

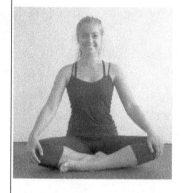

Energetic Benefits
It establishes a connection between the
physical body and beyond. It prepare the
spirit to receive the light.

Physical Benefits
It favors circulation in the lumbar spine
and the abdomen, and it rejuvenates the
spine.

Notes:

Baddha Konasana—Butterfly Pose

Skill: Beginner
Breath: Five
Drishti: Forward
Goal: To Open the Hips Naturally
Category: Sitting Position, Hip Opener,
Forward Fold

Technique
Sit on the floor and place the soles of the
feet together, opening the hips. Stretch the
spine with the top of the head up. Keep
the elbows at the sides of the body. Inhale
and lift while exhaling. Lower down.

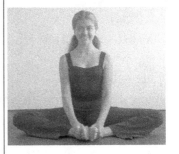

Modification
Sit on a blanket and open the legs in a
diamond shape.

Cues—Teaching Tips
Keep the hips on the floor and the knees
low. Keep the shoulders aligned in the back
with head and align them with the spine.

Energetic Benefits
It releases fears and soothes bad addictions.

Physical Benefits
It stimulates the blood in the pubic area,
cures urinary diseases, and activates the
kidneys, prostate, and bladder functions. It
prevents illness in the reproductive system.

Notes:

Padmasana—Lotus Pose

Skill: Intermediate
Breath: Five to Ten
Drishti: Forward
Goal: To Prepare for Meditation
Category: Sitting Position, Hip Opener

Technique
Sit down on the floor with crossed legs.
Bring the right heel and foot to the left
hip, and the left heel and foot to the right
hip. Sit tall and lengthen the spine.

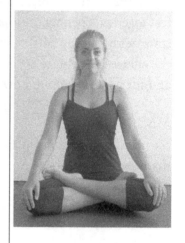

Modification
Stay in half lotus. Use blocks and blanket.

Cues—Teaching Tips
Keep the back straight and tall. Create
space in the abdomen. Maintain the
cervical spine and keep it aligned.

Energetic Benefits
It opens the mind and keeps one alert. It
invites prayer and enhances vitality.

Physical Benefits
It rejuvenates the pubic area, relaxes the
body, opens the hips, and strengthens the
knees.

Notes:

Parvatanasana—Hill Pose

Skill: Beginner
Breath: Five
Drishti: Down
Goal: To Develop Thorax and Restore Energy
Category: Sitting Position, Hip Openers

Technique
From Padmasana elongate the arms up
and clasp the fingers. Turn the palms
toward the ceiling.

Modification
Sit in Siddhasana and keep the arms
forward.

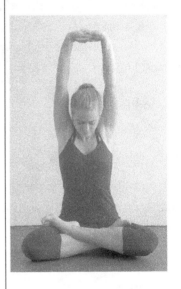

Cues—Teaching Tips
Lengthen the arms up and lower the chin.

Energetic Benefits
It improves the quality of expression and
brings courage and presence of mind.

Physical Benefits
It softens the rigidity of shoulders, opens
the hips, and strengthens the upper back.

Notes:

Marichyasana II—Wise Pose

Skill: Beginner
Breath: Five
Drishti: Ceiling
Goal: To Activate the Digestive System
Category: Sitting Position, Twist

Technique
From Dandasana bend one knee. On the same side, wrap the knees with one arm Hold the other hand behind you. Twist and look up.

Modification
Sit on a blanket and use a strap.

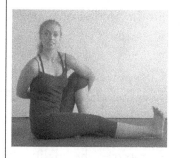

Cues—Teaching Tips
Spine lifted through the spine. Fully open the chest—leg on the floor active with flex foot.

Energetic Benefits
It brings tranquility, confidence, and good decisions.

Physical Benefits
It relieves pain from the neck, back, and hips. It tones the liver and spleen.

Notes:

Marichyasana III—Wise Pose

Skill: Beginner
Breath: Five
Drishti: Behind
Goal: To Stretch Hip Extensors
Category: Sitting Position, Twist

Technique
From Dandasana bend one knee and cross one leg over the other one, placing the foot on the floor. Place opposite elbow outside the knee and rotate the torso out and back.

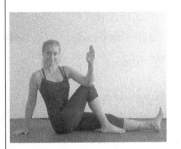

Modification
Keep the leg inside without crossing it. Place the opposite hand. Use a blanket.

Cues—Teaching Tips
Keep the back straight. Shoulders should be square with chest open. Ground the big toe on the floor.

Energetic Benefits
It creates a sense of responsibility and acceptance.

Physical Benefits
It helps lumbago and sciatica nerve. It increases the blood flow into internal organs, toning the liver and spleen.

Notes:

Single-Leg Stretch (An Exercise)

Skill: Beginner
Repetition: Six to Eight, Each Leg
Drishti: Navel
Breath: In Nose. out Mouth
Goal: To Strengthen Abdominal Muscles
Category: Abdominal Work from Pilates

Technique
Lying down, lift the head and bring one
leg to the chest. Extend the other leg out
on a diagonal. Switch sides.

Modification
Keep the head on the floor. Lift the legs
toward the ceiling.

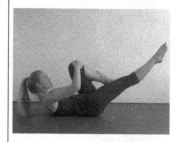

Cues—Teaching Tips
Keep the middle line active. Bring the
heels close to the gluteus. Press the
shoulder blades into the floor.

Energetic Benefits
It helps one let go of tension and stress.
It promotes self and offers serenity and
confidence.

Physical Benefits
It brings alignment and connection of the
center. It stabilizes and develops the pelvic
and lumbar region.

Notes:

Double-Leg Stretch (An Exercise)

Skill: Beginner
Repetition: Six to Eight
Drishti: Navel
Breath: In Nose, out Mouth
Goal: To Strengthen Abdominal Muscles
Category: Abdominal Work from Pilates

Technique
Lying down, lift the head and bring both legs
to the chest. Inhale and extend legs out on
a diagonal with arms over the head. Exhale
and fold the body to starting position.

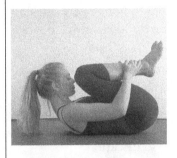

Modification
Keep the head on the floor and lengthen
the legs and arms toward the ceiling.

Cues—Teaching Tips
Hold the ankles. Press the shoulder blades
down. Use the core muscles to move the
limbs.

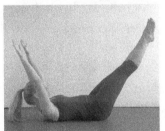

Energetic Benefits
It develops clearness of movement and
quality of expression. It releases resistance
and helps to think powerfully.

Physical Benefits
It strengthens and improves the endurance
of abdominal muscles. It teaches the body
to work in opposition and develops trunk
stabilization.

Notes:

Single Straight-Leg Stretch (An Exercise)

Skill: Beginner
Repetition: Six to Eight, Each Leg
Drishti: Navel
Breath: In Nose, out Mouth
Goal: To Strengthen Abdominal Muscles
Category: Abdominal Work from Pilates

Technique
Lying down, extend both legs up. Lift the chest and hold one ankle with both hands. Bring the leg toward the chest and the other one forward, bouncing two times. Switch legs.

Modification
Hold the leg behind the knee. Bend the knees. Keep the head on the floor.

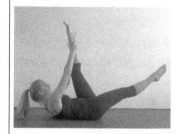

Cues—Teaching Tips
Don't move the body, just the legs. Work from the core muscles and keep the arms long.

Energetic Benefits
It activates the nervous system and helps one focus and concentrate. It balances memory skills.

Physical Benefits
It lengthens and reinforces natural strength of the legs. It improves alienation of the body and reinforces abdominal organs.

Notes:

Supta Baddha Konasana— Lying Butterfly Pose

Skill: Beginner
Breath: Five to Ten
Drishti: Ceiling, Eyes Closed
Goal: To Rest and Open Hips
Category: General Body Stretching

Technique
From Baddha Konasana lie back on the floor. Place arms over the head and form a box, holding the elbows. Rest peacefully.

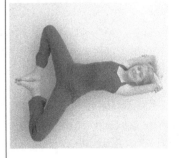

Modification
Keep the arms at the sides. Hold a strap and pull the ankles in. Keep the feet in Siddhasana pose. Use a blanket.

Cues—Teaching Tips
Flatten the spine down to the floor. Keep the soles of the feet together and breathe steadily.

Energetic Benefits
Tolerance resolves jealousy and self-judgment. It is good for shy people.

Physical Benefits
It expands the back, thorax, and neck—same effects as Baddha Konasana. It improves the heart and prevents lung disease.

Notes:

Supta Padangusthasana— Lying Big Toe Pose

Skill: Beginner
Breath: Five for Each Movement
Drishti: Forward and Side
Goal: To Reinforce Legs and Open the Hips
Category: General Body Stretches

Technique
Lying on the floor, bend one knee. Hold the big toe and lift the leg. Lift the chest and connect the forehead with the knee. Breathe for five. Keep opposite hand on the thigh. Open the leg to the side and breathe for five. Keep opposite hand on the hip. Return to the first position and breathe for one. Change leg.

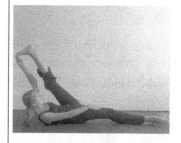

Modification
Use a strap and keep the chest on the floor. Use a blanket.

Cues—Teaching Tips
Relax the upper body and keep both legs active. Feel each movement differently.

Energetic Benefits
It releases emotional block and helps to set up goals. It brings presence to the moment.

Physical Benefits
It develops legs correctly. It activates the circulatory system and eliminates rigidity of hips.

Notes:

Anantasana—Side Leg Up Pose

Skill: Beginner
Breath: Five
Drishti: Forward
Goal: To Strengthen the Pelvis and the Hips
Category: General Body Stretch

Technique
Lying sideways, place the hand behind the
cervical spine. Bend the top knee, grab
the big toe, and extend the leg toward the
ceiling.

Modification
Keep the head down. Use a strap and
bend the bottom leg.

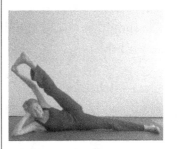

Cues—Teaching Tips
Avoid leaning back. Lengthen the back of
the neck and keep both legs active.

Energetic Benefits
It helps to make decisions and feel
comfort. It enhances general good health.

Physical Benefits
It lengthens the body, brings awareness,
and corrects posture.

Notes:

Sarvangasana—Shoulder Bridge Pose

Skill: Beginner
Breath: Five
Drishti: Toes
Goal: To Tone the Entire Body and Reinforce the Relation of Body to Mind
Category: Inversion

Technique
While lying down, lift both legs to the ceiling. Place hands on the lower back.

Modification
Use the wall and place a blanket under the shoulders. Bend the knees as you go toward the pose.

Cues—Teaching Tips
Keep the back straight with weight on the shoulders and tailbone forward. Keep legs perpendicular and together toward the ceiling.

Energetic Benefits
It brings joy, confidence, peace, and power of choice. It improves verbal communication.

Physical Benefits
It reinforces the arms, legs, and pelvic bone. It stimulates all the functions and systems of the body. It increases circulation.

Notes:

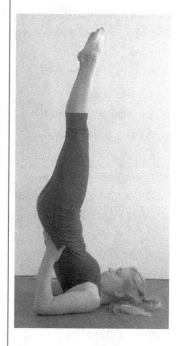

Halasana—Plough Pose

Skill: Beginner
Breath: Five
Drishti: Nose
Goal: To Rejuvenate the Spine, to Flex the Lower Back
Category: Inversion

Technique
From Sarvangasana lower the legs to the floor. Interlace fingers and extend the arms away.

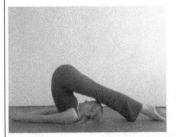

Modification
Lower one leg at a time. Support the lower back and place a block of chair behind to elevate the legs.

Cues—Teaching Tips
Keep the legs together with hips lifted. Maintain the weight on the shoulders and point the feet.

Energetic Benefits
It activates creativity and relaxes the mind. It brings awareness of emotional perception.

Physical Benefits
It helps the process of eliminating waste from the digestive track—it activates the thyroid and parathyroid glands. Remember to call the bandhas.

Notes

Chapter 7

Intermediate Asana

Standing Positions
1. Utthita Trikonasana
2. Parivrtta Trikonasana
3. Utthita Parsvakonasana
4. Parivrtta Parsvakonasana

Balance Positions
5. Natarajasana
6. Garudasana

Back Bends
7. Setu Bandhasana
8. Bhekasana
9. Dhanurasana

Sitting Positions, Forward Folds
10. Ardha Baddha Padma Paschimottanasana
11. Janu Sirsasana
12. Parivrtta Janu Sirsasana

Hip Openers
13. Virasana
14. Mulabandhasana
15. Yoga Mudrasana

Twists
16. Ardha Matsyendrasana
17. Bharadvajasana I
18. Malasana I

Abdominal Work
Pilates
    19. Crisscross
    20. Rolling Like A Ball
    21. The Saw

General Body Stretches
    22. Jathara Parivartanasana
    23. Parighasana
    24. Supta Virasana
    25. Matsyasana

Inversions
    26. Karnapidasana
    27. Sirsasana

Utthita Trikonasana—Triangle Pose

Skill: Intermediate
Breath: 5
Drishti: Thumb
Goal: To Strengthen the Spine and Legs
Category: Standing Position

Technique
From Tadasana open the legs apart, one foot out and the other in—arms out. Lean the body toward the front leg. Rotate the rib cage to the ceiling and extend the top arm up.

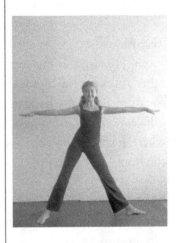

Modification
Bend the front knee a bit. Place a block behind the front foot. Keep the hand on the hip.

Cues—Teaching Tips
Open the chest and keep the top arm in line with the shoulder. Engage both legs.

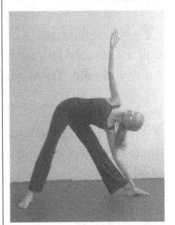

Energetic Benefits
It stabilizes the mind and maintains order and structure. It also obtains self-peace.

Physical Benefits
It tones all muscles of the body and stretches the spine. It releases tension from ankles and knees.

Notes:

Parivrtta Trikonasana— Revolved Triangle

Skill: Intermediate
Breath: Five
Drishti: Thumb
Goal: To Define Twist Movement in the Spine
Category: Standing Position, Twist

Technique
From Tadasana, bring one leg behind the other and keep the hips front in an internal rotation. Place the hands on the hips and inhale. Look up and exhale, leaning forward with flat spine. Twist the body to the side of the front leg. Extend the arms in line.

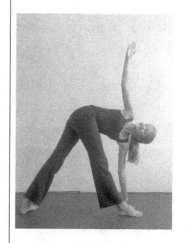

Modification
Keep the front knee bent, hand on the hip, and use a block.

Cues—Teaching Tips
Pull the sternum forward; the leg behind is active and solid. Try to look at the thumb.

Energetic Benefits
It brings peace and tranquility. It increases discipline and perseverance, and promotes good health.

Physical Benefits
It tones calf muscles and improves digestion. It rejuvenates the spine.

Notes:

Utthita Parsvakonasana — Extended Side Angle

Skill: Intermediate
Breath: Five
Drishti: Thumb
Goal: To Strengthen the Spine and Legs
Category: Standing Position

Technique
From Virabhadrasana II place the front hand behind the front knee and extend the arm behind the ear.

Modification
Use a block. Shorten the stand and cross the elbow on the thigh.

Cues—Teaching Tips
Use the back leg as a stabilizing tool. Look at the thumb as you rotate the rib cage up.

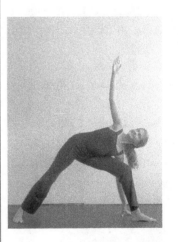

Energetic Benefits
It bring stability of the mind and security in your actions. It opens the heart to compassion and hope.

Physical Benefits
It cures and alleviates sciatica nerve, helps arthritis, and aids elimination.

Notes:

Parivrtta Parsvakonasana— Revolved Side Angle

Skill: Intermediate
Breath: Five
Drishti: Thumb
Goal: To Activate Digestion Function and Reinforce the Body
Category: Standing Position, Twist

Technique
From Virabhadrasana II turn the torso toward the front. Place opposite arm outside the front foot. Rotate the torso and lengthen the top arm.

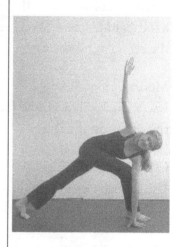

Modification
Place the back knee on the floor. Keep the hand inside the foot and keep the other hand on the hip.

Cues—Teaching Tips
Keep the hips square as possible and stretch the arms in opposition. Activate the back leg and maintain the lunge.

Energetic Benefits
It relieves anxiety and depression, and it enhances vitality of order and structure. It eliminates guilt, shame, and blame.

Physical Benefits
It increases circulation in the digestive track and helps abdominal organs, the spine, and legs.

Notes:

Natarajasana—Dancer Pose

Skill: Intermediate
Breath: Five
Drishti: Forward
Goal: To Promote Balance
Category: Standing Position, Balance

Technique
From Tadasana bend one knee and hold
the ankle. Find the balance, lean forward,
and kick the leg behind. Come out with
the same precision.

Modification
Use the wall for support. Lower the chest
toward the floor and use a strap.

Cues—Teaching Tips
Find the focal point, breathe deeply, and
activate the supporting leg.

Energetic Benefits
It establishes confidence and brings
acceptance, joy, and gratitude.

Physical Benefits
It expands the chest, benefits the vertebrae,
and brings elegance to the movement.

Notes:

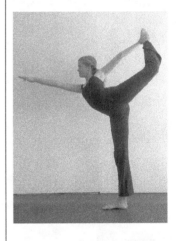

Garudasana—Eagle Pose

Skill: Intermediate
Breath: Five
Drishti: Forward
Goal: To Activate All the Joints
Category: Standing Position, Balance

Technique
From Tadasana, drop the hips and bend one leg on top of other. Clasp the ankles behind, cross the arms, and hold hands.

Modification
Place the top foot on a block. Keep elbows together and extend the hands up, breaking out the pose.

Cues—Teaching Tips
Bend the knees without leaning forward. Squeeze the joints into one each other and strengthen the internal muscles.

Energetic Benefits
It brings a new equilibrium, spontaneity in helping others, and self-confidence to let go of shame and blame.

Physical Benefits
It improves the health of joints and relieves the stiffness of shoulders.

Notes:

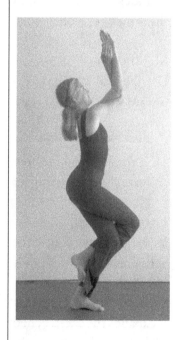

Setu Bandhasana—Bridge Pose

Skill: Intermediate
Breath: Five
Drishti: Tip of Nose or Ceiling
Goal: To Articulate the Spine and Prepare for Deeper Back Bends
Category: Back Bend

Technique
Lie down and bend the knees hip-width distance apart. Lift the hips and chest. Interlace the fingers and extend the knuckles of the fingers toward the heels. Tuck the chin in.

Modification
Use a block. Don't interlace fingers.

Cues—Teaching Tips
Keep the hips high and press the shoulders down. Keep the tailbone forward.

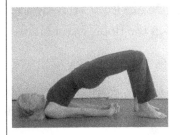

Energetic Benefits
It inspires emotional perception and helps one to let go of the past.

Physical Benefits
It removes stiffness from the back and brings flexibility to the spine as well as dorsal and lumbar areas.

Notes:

Bhekasana—Frog Pose

Skill: Intermediate
Breath: Five
Drishti: Forward
Goal: To Cure Deformities of Knees and Ankles
Category: Back Bend

Technique
Lie down, bend both knees, and hold the tip of the feet and try to lower them to the floor. Lift the chest up.

Modification
Do one leg at a time and keep the forehead on the floor. Use a blanket.

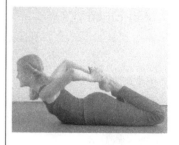

Cues—Teaching Tips
Try to lower the feet without lifting the knees off the floor—the elbows lift up.

Energetic Benefits
It opens the capacity of honoring yourself and strengthens your beliefs.

Physical Benefits
It firms and alleviates the knees, ankles, and heels. It benefits the abdominal organs as they are pressed strongly.

Notes:

Dhanurasana—Bow Pose

Skill: Intermediate
Breath: Five
Drishti: Forward—Three Eye
Goal: To Stretch the Whole Spine
Category: Back Bend

Technique
Lie down, bend both legs, and hold the ankles. Lift the legs and chest, kicking the legs behind.

Modification
Use a strap and place a blanket under the belly. Lift only the leg.

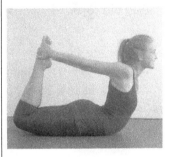

Cues—Teaching Tips
Keep the knees as close together as possible. Move in and out of the pose a few times. Kick the legs away from the shoulders.

Energetic Benefits
It brings courage and awareness. It releases feelings of shyness and guilt.

Physical Benefits
It brings elasticity, and stretches and tones the whole spine. It tones the abdominal organs.

Notes:

Ardha Baddha Padma Paschimottanasana—Half Lotus

Skill: Intermediate
Breath: 5
Drishti: Big Toe
Goal: To Stretch the Knees and Ankles
Category: Sitting Pose, Forward Folds

Technique
From Dandasana bend one knee and place the ankle near the groin. Bend the opposite arm behind you and hold the foot. Fold forward.

Modification
Grab the foot with same side hand or practice Janu Sirsasana. Use the strap and sit on a blanket. Place a block under the bended knee.

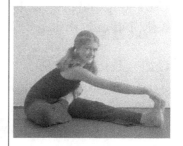

Cues—Teaching Tips
Lengthen forward from the lower back and maintain the shoulders and shoulder blades on place.

Energetic Benefits
Let go of resistance and resentment. Open doors to a bigger perception.

Physical Benefits
It brings flexibility to the knees and shoulders, and stimulates the digestive system.

Notes:

Janu Sirsasana—Head-to-Knee Fold

Skill: Intermediate
Breath: Five
Drishti: Forward to Big Toe
Goal: To Activate an Internal Digestive Track and Stretch the Spine
Category: Sitting Pose, Forward Fold

Technique
From Dandasana bend one knee as a tree pose. Lengthen the spine tall and bend forward to the long leg in front of you.

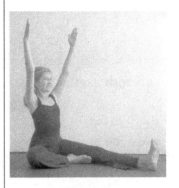

Modification
Use a strap. Bend the knee in front. Place a block under the bended knee and sit down on a blanket.

Cues—Teaching Tips
Lengthen from the lower back and lengthen the crown of the head toward the big toe.

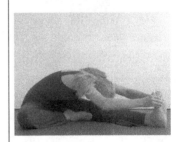

Energetic Benefits
It keeps the heart open for the well-being. It helps one find pleasure in actions and discover peace of mind.

Physical Benefits
It activates the kidneys and tones the internal organs, including the liver and spleen. It rejuvenates the spine and increases blood flow in the pubic area.

Notes:

Parivrtta Janu Sirsasana— Revolved Head-to-Knee Fold

Skill: Intermediate
Breath: Five
Drishti: Forward to Ceiling
Goal: To Rejuvenate the Spine
Category: Sitting Position, Twist

Technique
From Janu Sirsasana extend the long leg to the side. Side bend and grab the foot with both hands. Stretch the spine.

Modification
Side bend and keep the top hand on the hip. Use a blanket, strap, and block under the elbow.

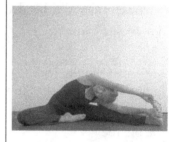

Cues—Teaching Tips
Rotate the rib cage. Maintain steady the strength of legs and sit bones.

Energetic Benefits
It enhances self-esteem, motivation, and freedom for the yoga practice.
Physical Benefits
It activates circulation in the spine, rejuvenating the nerves and vertebras, and fully expanding the internal organs.

Notes:

Virasana—Hero Pose

Skill: Intermediate
Breath: Five
Drishti: Forward
Goal: To Correct Back Deformities and Heal the Knees
Category: Sitting Position, Hip Opener

Technique
From kneeling position, separate the calf apart and sit down in between the legs. Keep the knees together and place hands on tops of knees and close the eyes.

Modification
Sit down on a block or folded blanket.

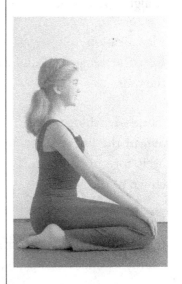

Cues—Teaching Tips
Keep the back straight, lower the chin, and press the toes down.

Energetic Benefits
It brings serenity and relaxation of mind, develops patience and tolerance, and finds pleasures in daily actions.

Physical Benefits
It strengthens the ankles, cures rheumatoid knee problems, and reduces calcium deposits from the heels.

Notes:

Mulabandhasana—Squat Pose

Skill: Intermediate
Breath: Five
Drishti: Forward
Goal: To Reinforce the Pelvic Floor Muscles and Promote Balance
Category: Hip Opener

Technique
From Baddha Konasana, place the feet near the perineum and lift up with straight spine. Place hands in Namaste.

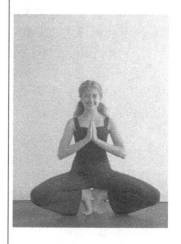

Modification
Keep the feet apart, lean forward, and use the wall.

Cues—Teaching Tips
Spread the knees apart and squeeze the heels together and up. Lift through the crown of the head.

Energetic Benefits
It gives security, confidence, and vitality. It eliminates jealousy and opens consciousness.
Physical Benefits
It is good for menstrual disease, brings balance, and stabilizes motion in the body.

Notes:

Yoga Mudrasana—Seal Pose

Skill: Intermediate
Breath: Five
Drishti: Eyes Close
Goal: To Seal the Practice and Invite Prayer
Category: Sitting Position, Hip Opener

Technique
From Padmasana hold the elbows behind the back and lower the back and head forward.

Modification
Place blocks under the knees and extend the arms behind.

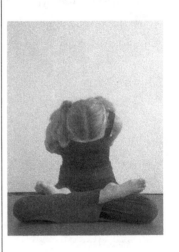

Cues—Teaching Tips
Bring the head all the way to the floor. Express gratitude and press the knees down.

Energetic Benefits
It soothes and comforts, and promotes stress-free living. It increases self-love and intuition for right decisions.
Physical Benefits
It expands the thorax and alleviates constipation. It aids digestion and increases movement of the shoulders.

Notes:

Ardha Matsyendrasana—Twist Pose

Skill: Intermediate
Breath: Five
Drishti: Back
Goal: To Stretch the Spine in Rotation
Category: Sitting Position, Twist

Technique
From Dandasana cross one leg on top of the other. Slice the other leg behind. With the opposite hand hold the top knee (elbow) and twist tall and behind.

Modification
Do Marichyasana III. Hold the knee with the hand. Use a blanket.

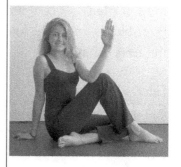

Cues—Teaching Tips
Keep the spine tall and push down with the big toe. Open the chest.

Energetic Benefits
It encourages courage, braveness, and security. It opens others to new ideas for the future.

Physical Benefits
It favors the digestive and reproductive organs. It stretches the spine and the upper thoracic area.

Notes:

Bharadvajasana I—Sage Pose

Skill: Intermediate
Breath: Five
Drishti: Ceiling
Goal: To Repair the Dorsal and Lumbar Region
Category: Sitting Position, Twist

Technique
From Dandasana bend the knees to one side, keeping the ankles together. Bend the opposite side arm and hold the elbow behind the back. Place same side arm to the top knee. Twist and look up.

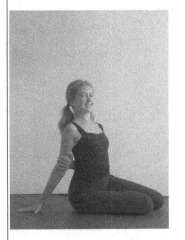

Modification
Keep the arm on the back and twist both sides, Separate the legs and sit down on a blanket.

Cues—Teaching Tips
Press the back elbow to the top area of the kidneys and squeeze the hips together.

Energetic Benefits
It corrects bad eating habits, develops faith and devotion, and helps with communication.
Physical Benefits
It rejuvenates the dorsal area, helps with arthritis, and activates the endocrine system.

Notes:

Malasana—Garland Pose

Skill: Intermediate
Breath: Five
Drishti: Ceiling
Goal: To Tone the Spine
Category: Sitting Position, Twist

Technique
From Tadasana separate the feet hip-width distance and squat down. Turn the body to one side. Keep the internal rotation of both shoulders and clasp the hands behind the back and knee.

Modification
Sit down and use a block and strap to hold hands or keep the hands on the floor front and back of side knee.

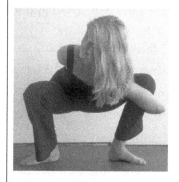

Cues—Teaching Tips
Open the chest and squeeze the knees apart. Lift the spine tall and look up.

Energetic Benefits
It helps to make good decisions and allows one to find security and confidence for what he or she wants.
Physical Benefits
It reinforces ankles, knees, and shoulders. It tones the spine, improves digestion, and cures disorders in the liver, spleen, and pancreas.

Notes:

Crisscross (An Exercise)

Skill: Intermediate
Repetition: Six to Eight, Each Leg
Drishti: Elbow Behind
Breath: In Nose, out Mouth
Goal: To Strengthen Abdominal Muscles
Category: Abdominal Work from Pilates

Technique
Lie down and bring hands behind the head. Lift the chest and move the legs as a single-leg stretch, guiding the elbow to the opposite knee.

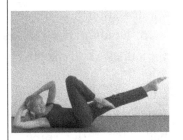

Modification
Place feet on the floor and lift the torso to find opposite elbow to knee. Rest each time.

Cues—Teaching Tips
Twist from the side and avoid turning the neck. Look to back elbow and move from the core muscles. Press the shoulder blades down toward the floor.

Energetic Benefits
It challenges the rotation, develops trunk stabilization, and improves and reinforces abdominal muscles.

Physical Benefits
It quiets the mind with confidence, faith, and intuition.

Notes:

Rolling Like a Ball (An Exercise)

Skill: Intermediate
Repetition: Six through Eight
Drishti: Belly
Breath: In Nose. out Mouth
Goal: To Strengthen Abdominal Muscles
Category: Abdominal Work from Pilates

Technique
Bend the knees into your body and form
a little ball. Place hands on ankles and roll
back and forth.

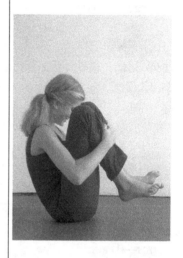

Modification
Place hands under the knees and open
the ankles. Hold the pose without rolling.

Cues—Teaching Tips
Relax the shoulders and look at the
belly. Press the spine down through
the movement and look to your belly
throughout the movement.

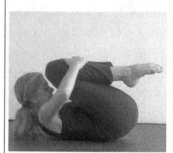

Energetic Benefits
It brings presence, faith, and confidence
in your movement.

Physical Benefits

It massages and stimulates the spine. It
brings back vitality and cures back pain.

Notes:

The Saw (An Exercise)

Skill: Intermediate
Repetition: Six to Eight, Each Leg
Drishti: Hand Behind
Breath: Inhale in Nose, Exhale from Mouth
Goal: To Teach Straight and C-Curve Back
Category: Abdominal Work from Pilates

Technique
Sit on the floor with legs apart and straight back. Rotate the torso to one side and fold over the leg in a C curve, stretching the arms in opposition. Lift and return to the starting position with the back straight.

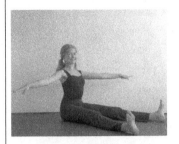

Modification
Bend knees with feet on the floor. In the same movement, place the back of the hand on the floor and head toward the knee.

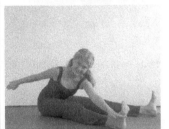

Cues—Teaching Tips
Clear the movement with the breath. Keep the sit bones on the floor and your feet in flex position.
Energetic Benefits
It gives self-acceptance and self-respect. It allows one to let go of shame and guilt.

Physical Benefits
It extends the spine in rotation, improves respiration patterns, and strengthens the muscles in the back.

Notes:

Jathara Parivartanasana— Rolling Stomach Twist

Skill: Intermediate
Breath: Five
Drishti: Ceiling
Goal: To Help Digestion and Lengthens the Legs
Category: General Body Stretches, Twist

Technique
Lying down, open the arms in a cross position with legs to the ceiling. Squeeze the legs and lower them to one side, trying to get the opposite shoulder down.

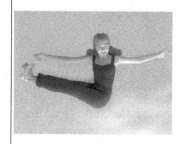

Modification
Place a blanket under the lower back and practice regular spinal twist.

Cues—Teaching Tips
Look at the ceiling. Keep your knees and ankles together. Reach the hand toward the toes.

Energetic Benefits
It helps one to process the experiences of life, and it awakens vulnerability and surrender with illumination and self-respect.

Physical Benefits
It tones the spleen, liver, and pancreas. It strengthens the lower back and hips.

Notes:

Parighasana—Bar Pose

Skill: Intermediate
Breath: Five
Drishti: Forward
Goal: To Strengthen the Sides of the Body and the Spine
Category: General Body Stretch, Side Bend

Technique
From a kneeling position, extend one leg to the side with one foot out. Bend over the leg with the opposite arm over the ear.

Modification
Place a blanket under the bended knee. Bend the knee and keep the hand on the hip with a block.

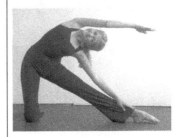

Cues—Teaching Tips
Keep the knee strong and the foot out. Press down with the feet. Try to reach long with both arms.

Energetic Benefits
It gives personal power, responsibility, and control of energy.

Physical Benefits
It stretches the muscles of the pelvis, extending the side of the abdomen. It helps rigidity of the back and brings sense of alignment.

Notes:

Supta Virasana—Lying-Down Hero

Skill: Intermediate
Breath: Five
Drishti: Ceiling
Goal: To Lengthen the Spine and Abdominal Organs
Category: General Body Stretch, Hip Opener

Technique
From Virasana, lie on your back, arms over your head. Hold the elbows.

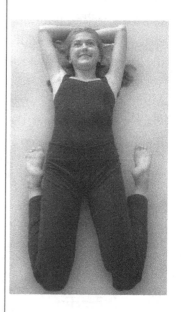

Modification
Stay in your elbows. Place a block under your head and lower back. Use a blanket and separate the knees.

Cues—Teaching Tips
Keep the shoulder blades down and lower the rib cage. Keep your knees together.

Energetic Benefits
It helps to express desires and invites communication, confidence, and security.

Physical Benefits
It lengthens abdominal organs, muscles of the pelvis, and the quads. It improves the health of the legs.

Notes

Matsyasana—Fish Pose

Skill: Intermediate
Breath: Five
Drishti: Behind
Goal: To Counteract Heaviness of Shoulders
Category: General Body Stretch, Back Bend

Technique
From lying down, arch your back and keep the weight on top of the head and in the elbows. Legs are long and together with straight feet.

Modification
Place a block under the head. Back off the arch.

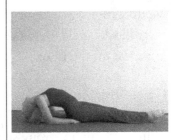

Cues—Teaching Tips
Lengthen the body in opposition from head to toes. Squeeze the hips and extend the ankles.

Energetic Benefits
It increases the power of speech and allows one to be fearless and accept and let go of worries.

Physical Benefits
It improve the respiratory and endocrine systems.

Notes:

Karnapidasana—Knees to Ear Pose

Skill: Intermediate
Breath: Five
Drishti: Upward
Goal: To Rest the Body and Cure Ear Disease
Category: Inversion

Technique
From Halasana bend the knees and rest them on the floor beside the ears. Interlace the fingers and lengthen the arms in opposition.

Modification
Place blocks under the knees and keep the arms flat on the floor.

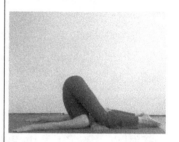

Cues—Teaching Tips
Keep the spine perpendicular to the ceiling. Maintain strong shoulders.

Energetic Benefits
It promotes happiness, opens a vision of abundance, and empowers self-esteem.

Physical Benefits
It rests the heart and lungs, and it stretches the spine completely.

Notes:

Sirsasana—Head Stand

Skill: Intermediate
Breath: Ten
Drishti: Behind
Goal: To Balance the Body and Open to Inner Light
Category: Inversion

Technique
From Down Gog place elbows on the floor. Walk the feet near the body. Lift one leg and the other to an upside-down position.

Modification
Keep the position of preparation. Practice on the wall.

Cues—Teaching Tips
Keep the weight on your shoulders and the legs strong and together.

Energetic Benefits
It helps one to let go of judgment and find illumination and strength in self-belief.

Physical Benefits
It activates pineal and pituitary glands, and it keeps the body warm. It soothes the nervous system.

Notes:

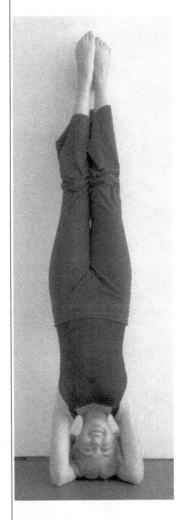

Chapter 8

Advanced Asana

Standing Positions
1. Parsvottanasana
2. Anjaneyasana
3. Virabhadrasana II
4. Ardha Chandrasana V

Balance Positions
5. Ardha Chandrasana
6. Urdhva Prasarita Eka Padasana

Back Bends
7. Purvottanasana
8. Urdhva Dhanurasana
9. Ustrasana

Sitting Positions
Forward Folds
10. Triang Mukhaikapada Paschimottanasana
11. Krounchasana
12. Navasana
13. Marichyasana I

Hip Openers
14. Eka Pada Rajakapotasana
15. Upavistha Konasana
16. Gomukhasana

Twists
17. Parivrtta Utkatasana

18. Parivrtta Anjaneyasana

Arm Balances
19. Bakasana
20. Tolasana
21. Vasisthasana

Abdominal Work
Pilates
22. Front and Back
23. Up and Down
24. Shoulder Bridge
25. Swan Dive

General Body Stretches
26. Hanumanasana
27. Kurmasana
28. Supta Parivrtta Garudasana

Inversion
29. Adho Mukha Vrksasana

Savasana: Final Relaxation

Parsvottanasana—Pyramid

Skill: Advanced
Breath: Five
Drishti: Knee and Big Toe
Goal: To Stretch the Legs and Clear the Respiratory System
Category: Standing Position

Technique
From Tadasana bring one leg back and keep an internal rotation of the hips. Place hands in Namaste on the back. Bend forward to connect the forehead with your knee.

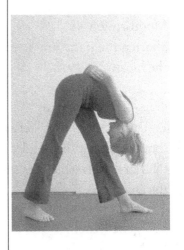

Modification
Bend the front knee or practice on the wall.

Cues—Teaching Tips
Breathe to the bottom of the lungs. Keep the legs still and strong.

Energetic Benefits
It opens the mind to change and activates creativity.

Physical Benefits
It keeps the hips flexible and stretches the legs. It corrects round shoulders and tones internal organs.

Notes:

Virabhadrasana II—Warrior II

Skill: Advanced
Breath: Five
Drishti: Front Fingertips
Goal: To Stretch the Legs, Arms, and Torso
Category: Standing Position

Technique
From Virabhadrasana I rotate the hips to
an external rotation, lengthen the arms in
a cross, look forward, and stretch.

Modification
Shorten the stand and keep the hands on
the hips.

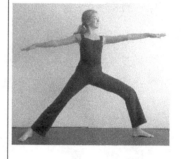

Cues—Teaching Tips
Find the opposition between knee and
shoulder. Keep the bended leg parallel to
the floor. Relax the toes and knee under
the ankle.

Energetic Benefits
It develops security and freedom of
movement, and it helps you to move
forward.

Physical Benefits
It reinforces leg muscles and establishes
power on the pelvic floor. It aligns the
arms, correcting shoulders.

Notes:

Anjaneyasana—Crescent Lunge

Skill: Advanced
Breath: Five
Drishti: Forward
Goal: To Master Body Mobility
Category: Standing Position

Technique
From Adho Mukha Svanasana bring one leg forward and stay in the ball of the back foot. Go into a lunge, raise the arms, interlace fingers, and point up with the index finger.

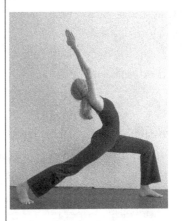

Modification
Keep the back knee on the floor, with arms separate.

Cues—Teaching Tips
Concentrate on stretching the arms up while the pelvis goes down. Place tailbone forward and use the back leg as stabilizer.

Energetic Benefits
It helps you to surrender and let go of judging and controlling others.

Physical Benefits
It rejuvenates the muscles, improves balance, and brings freedom of the body.

Notes:

Ardha Chandrasana V—Revolved Warrior

Skill: Advanced
Breath: Three
Drishti: Ceiling
Goal: To Flex the Spine and Prepare for Deeper Back Bends
Category: Standing Position, Back Bend

Technique
From Virabhadrasana II lengthen the
back arm toward the ankle and extend the
front arm toward the ceiling and behind.

Modification
Keep the back of the hand on the hips and
moderate the back bend.

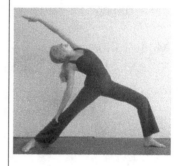

Cues—Teaching Tips
Reach the back of the hand near the ankle
and maintain the position of the legs.

Energetic Benefits
It develops hope, faith, and acceptance.

Physical Benefits
It improves heart circulation, reinforces
leg muscles, and masters the stand of
Virabhadrasana II.

Notes:

Ardha Chandrasana—Half Moon Pose

Skill: Advanced
Breath: Five
Drishti: Ceiling
Goal: To Improve Balance and Cure Hips and Back
Category: Standing Position, Balance

Technique
From Tadasana lift one leg behind at the level of the hip, rotate the rib cage to the side, and extend the arm up.

Modification
Practice the pose on the wall with a block.

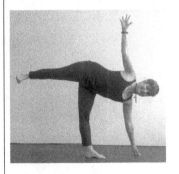

Cues—Teaching Tips
Flex the foot and create distance between the floor and the chest. Stay strong with the four limbs.

Energetic Benefits
It brings self–respect, eliminates guilt and blame, and helps to stay present in the moment.
Physical Benefits
It improves balance and reinforces the joints. It helps gastric disorders.

Notes:

Urdhva Prasarita Eka Padasana —One Leg Up

Skill: Advanced
Breath: Five
Drishti: Knee
Goal: To Promote Balance and Stabilization
Category: Standing Position, Balance

Technique
From Uttanasana bend one leg and place the knee toward the ceiling, then lengthen the full leg up to the ceiling. Keep the head near the supporting knee. With the opposite hand hold the ankle.

Modification
Keep both hands on the floor or on the block. Practice near the wall.

Cues—Teaching Tips
Point the leg straight to the ceiling. Look for opposition between the head and foot.

Energetic Benefits
It stimulates emotional health and creates pleasure in simple things.
Physical Benefits
It reduces fat from the waistline, stabilizes the mind, and reinforces the leg muscles and back.

Notes:

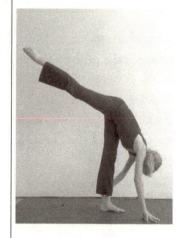

Purvottanasana—East Stretch

Skill: Advanced
Breath: Five
Drishti: Behind
Goal: To Lengthen the Body
Category: Back Bend

Technique
From Dandasana place the hands behind the hips with fingers toward the backs of the heels. Flatten the feet and lift the hips, lengthening the body from head to toes.

Modification
Bend the knees and come up to the table pose.

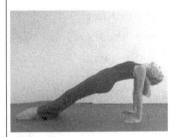

Cues—Teaching Tips
Use the biceps and strength of the abdomen. Rotate inner thighs and squeeze hips hard. Keep the feet together.

Energetic Benefits
It brings peace and balance and helps you to let go of bitterness.
Physical Benefits
It strengthens the hips and ankles. It improves shoulders' flexibility and fully expands the chest.

Notes:

Urdhva Dhanurasana—Wheel Stretch

Skill: Advanced
Breath: Five
Drishti: Behind
Goal: To Bring Elasticity to the Spine
Category: Back Bend

Technique
From Setu Bandhasana, rotate the arms and place the hands under the shoulders. Lift the back and straighten the arms, arching the back.

Modification
Keep the head on the floor in Setu Bandhasana.

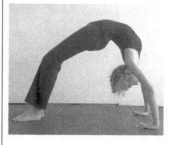

Cues—Teaching Tips
Lift the hips and maintain the hands under the shoulders. Maintain the feet distance apart.

Energetic Benefits
It promotes stillness and emotional stability. It deepens a sense of security and confidence.

Physical Benefits
It cures problems of the vertebrae. It reinforces the whole body and maintains the digestive and respiratory systems, keeping them active and healthy.

Notes:

Ustrasana—Camel Pose

Skill: Advanced
Breath: Five
Drishti: Up
Goal: To Tone the Spine
Category: Back Bend

Technique
From a kneeling position, place hands behind the back. Hold the ankles and stretch the back.

Modification
Keep the hands on the hips. Use a blanket.

Cues—Teaching Tips
Keep knees hip-width distance apart. Lift the chest, moving hips forward on tops of knees.

Energetic Benefits
It helps you to let go of repression, resentment, and disappointment. It brings peace and tranquility.

Physical Benefits
It corrects dropped shoulders and hunched back. It tones the whole spine and brings elasticity to the back. It improves the respiratory system.

Notes:

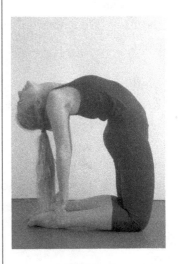

Triang Mukhaikapada Paschimottanasana—Ankle Behind Fold

Skill: Advanced
Breath: Five
Drishti: Down
Goal: To Stretch Knees, Ankles, and Hips
Category: Forward Fold

Technique
From Dandasana bend one knee toward the back. Do a forward fold toward the front.

Modification
Keep the leg in Janu Sirsasana position. Use a blanket.

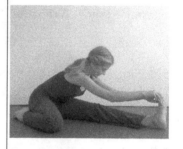

Cues—Teaching Tips
Lower the opposite hip down. Keep the front foot flexed and lengthen the spine to the leg.

Energetic Benefits
It teaches you to honor all things.

Physical Benefits
It reduces swelling legs. It activates the internal organs.

Notes:

Krounchasana—Heron Pose

Skill: Advanced
Breath: Five
Drishti: Big Toe
Goal: To Completely Extend the Leg Muscles
Category: Sitting Pose

Technique
From Triang Mukhaikapada Paschimottanasana or other sitting pose, lift the extended leg to the ceiling. Hold the foot or ankle. Keep the shoulder blades and shoulders in their sockets.

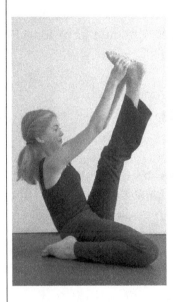

Modification
Use a strap or blanket while bending the top knee. Use other position of the back leg.

Cues—Teaching Tips
Keep the back straight and tall with the chest fully open. Elongate the leg from the hip and maintain the toes at eye level.

Energetic Benefits
It brings order and structure in the actions. It opens new relationships to unconditional love.

Physical Benefits
It completely extends the legs, tendons, ligaments, and bones. It rejuvenates the abdomen muscles.

Notes:

Navasana—Boat Pose

Skill: Advanced
Breath: Five
Drishti: Toes
Goal: To Strengthen the Back and Stabilize the Body
Category: Sitting Pose

Technique
From Dandasana extend both legs, forming a V position of the body with legs up and arms long toward the feet. Hold and balance.

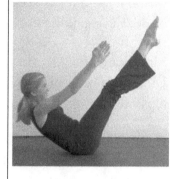

Modification
Sit on a blanket. Bend and hold the backs of the knees.

Cues—Teaching Tips
Elongate the legs and spine. Stretch the ankles, feet, and fingers. Use the muscles of the upper back.

Energetic Benefits
It reinforces self-esteem, self-respect, and honor. It motivates the practice.
Physical Benefits
It activates the internal organs, including liver, gallbladder, and spleen. The back becomes strong.

Notes:

Marichyasana I—Sage Pose

Skill: Advanced
Breath: Five
Drishti: Down
Goal: To Improve Digestion and Flexibility of the Spine
Category: Forward Fold

Technique
From Dandasana bend one knee to the level of the other knee. Interlace the hands behind and bend forward.

Modification
Use a blanket and strap. Push with the same arms to conquer the pose down.

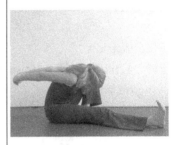

Cues—Teaching Tips
Keep the length from the lumbar spine. Use the breath to deepen the pose.

Energetic Benefits
It helps to discover abundance and pleasure in all your daily actions.

Physical Benefits
It provides an extreme contraction of the abdominal organs to improve digestion.

Notes:

Eka Pada Rajakapotasana—Pigeon Pose

Skill: Advanced
Breath: Five
Drishti: Up and Down
Goal: To Open and Strengthen the Hips
Category: Hip Opener

Technique
From Adho Mukha Svanasana, bend one knee and place the foot forward in pigeon position. Lower the body forward and relax.

Modification
Place a blanket. Do supine pigeon (while lying on your back).

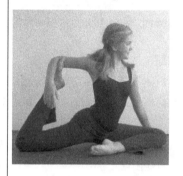

Cues—Teaching Tips
Square the hips. Keep the leg behind long and strong. Relax the stomach.

Energetic Benefits
It illuminates new paths and eliminates bad addictions. It helps you sense responsibilities.

Physical Benefits
It activates circulation in the pubic area. Urinary system and adrenal glands improve.

Notes:

Upavistha Konasana—Straddle

Skill: Advanced
Breath: Five
Drishti: Down
Goal: To Heal the Whole Body
Category: Hip Opener

Technique
From Dandasana spread out the legs. Hold the sides of the feet and fold forward.

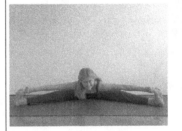

Modification
Sit on a blanket. Bend the knees slightly and try to move forward.

Cues—Teaching Tips
Keep the legs strong and long. Reach the chin to the floor. Keep feet in a flexed position.

Energetic Benefits
It liberates the body. It brings relaxation, prosperity, and patience.

Physical Benefits
It lengthens the leg muscles and the whole back. It prevents sciatica disorders and inguinal hernias. It is good for symptoms of menstrual periods.

Notes:

Gomukhasana—Cow Pose

Skill: Advanced
Breath: Five
Drishti: Forward
Goal: To Bring Elasticity to Leg Muscles
Category: Hip Opener

Technique
From a kneeling position, cross one leg over the other and place the top ankle behind. Lengthen the arm behind and capture the other hand in the middle of the back.

Modification
Sit on the sitting bones, knee over knee. Practice Garudasana arms.

Cues—Teaching Tips
Lengthen the spine and squeeze the legs. Lift the neck with shoulders in place.

Energetic Benefits
It brings pleasure to the practice, stability in the path, and capacity to help others.

Physical Benefits
It is the best pose for leg cramps. It opens the chest and the dorsal area.

Notes:

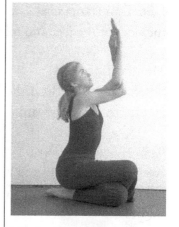

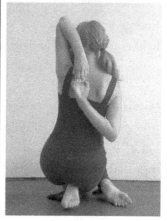

Parivrtta Utkatasana—Revolved Chair

Skill: Advanced
Breath: Five
Drishti: Sideways
Goal: To Develop Leg Muscles
Category: Standing Position, Twist

Technique
From Utkatasana, place hands in Namaste.
Lower the hips and twist the torso.

Modifications
Keep legs hip-width distance apart and
use a block for an easy twist.

Cues—Teaching Tips
Keep the hips and knees square, and focus
on twisting from the rib cage. Shoulders
remain in one line. The breast bone moves
forward. Keep hands in the middle of the
chest.

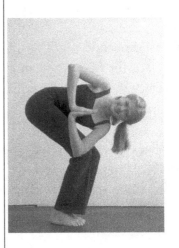

Energetic Benefits
It opens you to new projects, ambitions,
and goals.

Physical Benefits
It massages the internal organs, allowing
good function of the digestive track. It is
great for digestion.

Notes:

Parivrtta Anjaneyasana—Revolved Lunge

Skill: Advanced
Breath: Five
Drishti: Sideways
Goal: To Generate Movement with Alignment in the Body
Category: Standing Position, Twist

Technique
From Anjaneyasana place the hands in Namaste. Twist the body toward the side of the front knee.

Modification
Place the back knee on the floor. Use a block to lengthen the arms and extend the arms in opposition.

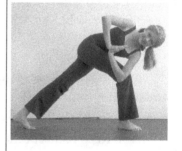

Cues—Teaching Tips
Keep your attention on the back leg, reaching the heel down. Twist from the rib cage, keeping the hands in the middle of the chest.

Energetic Benefits
It brings determination, stability, and freedom.

Physical Benefits
It keeps the body strong, benefits internal organs, and helps the body's mobility.

Notes:

Bakasana—Crane Pose

Skill: Advanced
Breath: Five
Drishti: Forward
Goal: To Manage the Balance and Weight of the Body
Category: Arm Balance

Technique
From Adho Mukha Svanasana, place the knees under the armpits, lean forward, and lift one leg, following the other. Balance and try to keep the arms straight.

Modification
Place the feet on a block and feel the sensation of being in the pose.

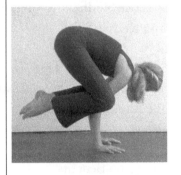

Cues—Teaching Tips
Lift the hips and keep the feet tall, keeping feet together and arms straight.

Energetic Benefits
It encourages practice and self-liberation.

Physical Benefits
It strengthens the wrist and abdominal muscles. It reinforces the whole body and promotes balance.

Notes:

Tolasana—Scale Pose

Skill: Advanced
Breath: Ten
Drishti: Forward
Goal: To Hold the Body off the Floor
Category: Arm Balance, Hip Opener

Technique
From Padmasana place the hands flat on the floor on either side of the body. Lift off and balance high.

Modification
Practice Siddhasana. Sit down on a block and feel the pose.

Cues—Teaching Tips
Focus and keep the spine straight. Lower the shoulder blades and lift from the pelvis.

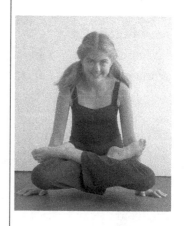

Energetic Benefits
It awakens self-value and activates purpose and intention.

Physical Benefits
It strengthens the wrists, promotes balance, and reinforces the pelvic floor muscles.

Notes:

Vasisthasana—Side Plank

Skill: Advanced
Breath: Five
Drishti: Forward
Goal: To Strengthen the Body on a Side Plane
Category: Arm Balance

Technique
From Plank position or Adho Mukha Svanasana, place one hand under the chest. Turn the body sideways. Keep one ankle over the other. Lengthen the top arm and find a vertical line with both arms.

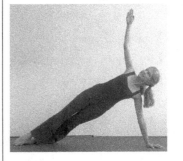

Modification
Place the bottom knee on the floor. Keep the top arm on the hip. Use a blanket.

Cues—Teaching Tips
Stretch the body from the head to the toes. Lift from the hips and strengthen the back muscles.

Energetic Benefits
It stimulates spontaneity and reinforces the heart and emotional perception.

Physical Benefits
It lengthens the body and reinforces the wrists, legs, and abdominal and lumbar region.

Notes:

Front and Back (An Exercise)

Skill: Advanced
Repetition: Six to Eight, Each Leg
Drishti: Forward
Breath: In Nose, out Mouth
Goal: To Lengthen and Reinforce the Legs
Category: Abdominal Work from Pilates

Technique
Lying down sideways, lift and kick the leg forward and back.

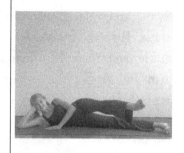

Modification
Lie down completely on the floor and bend the bottom leg.

Cues—Teaching Tips
Keep the pelvis still, move only the leg from the hip, and relax the ankles and toes.

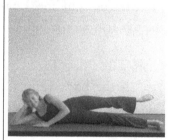

Energetic Benefits
It helps you to respond well to life.

Physical Benefits
It tones the thighs, hips, and abdomen. It strengthens the lower back and brings balance.

Notes:

Up and Down (An Exercise)

Skill: Advanced
Repetition: Five, Each Leg
Drishti: Corner of a Room
Breath: In Nose, out Mouth
Goal: To Strengthen Abdominal Muscles
Category: Abdominal Work from Pilates

Technique
Lying down sideways, rotate the top leg out. Lift it straight to the ceiling and lower.

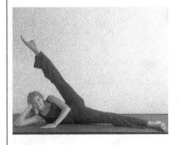

Modification
Lie down completely on the floor. Bend the bottom leg.

Cues—Teaching Tips
Keep the pelvis still and reach long with the legs. Touch the heels when they meet together and work energetically.

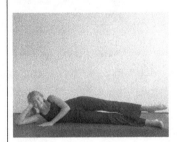

Energetic Benefits
It brings joy and allows you to move forward.

Physical Benefits
It lengthens and tones the thighs, hips, and abdominal muscles. It strengthens the lower back and promotes balance.

Notes:

Shoulder Bridge (An Exercise)

Skill: Intermediate
Repetition: Five Kicks, Each Leg
Drishti: Ceiling
Breath: In Nose, out Mouth
Goal: To Strengthen Abdominal Muscles
and the Hips
Category: Abdominal Work from Pilates

Technique
Lying down on bride position, bend one
knee and lengthen the leg to the ceiling.
Vigorously lower and lift the straight leg
five times.

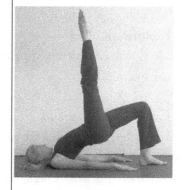

Modification
Keep the back flat on the floor as you
move the legs.

Cues—Teaching Tips
Keep the hips strong and don't let the hips
move up and down. Reach long through
the leg. Press with the shoulders hard and
head down to the mat.

Energetic Benefits
It organizes the thoughts and actions for
the day. It makes you notice the progress
in the practice.

Physical Benefits
It endures the whole body, reinforces the
abdominal muscles, and stabilizes the hips.

Notes:

Swan Dive (An Exercise)

Skill: Advanced
Repetition: Three to Five
Drishti: Forward
Breath: In Nose, out Mouth
Goal: To Strengthen Upper Back Muscles
Category: Abdominal Work from Pilates

Technique
Lie in a prone position. Place the hands under the shoulders and elbows, pointing toward the hips. Lift and lower the upper body, keeping the legs together.

Modification
Do basic spine extension with legs separated.

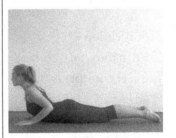

Cues—Teaching Tips
Keep the hips on the floor. Lift through the crown of the head. Keep the fingers together.

Energetic Benefits
It promotes decision, strength, balance, and generosity.

Physical Benefits
It stretches the abdominal muscles and neck, lengthening the spine in extension.

Notes:

Hanumanasana—Splits

Skill: Advanced
Breath: Five to Ten
Drishti: Forward
Goal: To Cure Leg Deformities
Category: General Body Stretches

Technique
From a kneeling position, place the hands in front of the knees, stretch, and lengthen the front leg forward and the back leg back. Lower the pelvis until it touches the floor. Lift and straighten the arms up.

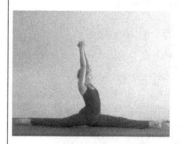

Modification
Keep hands on the blocks and lower as you feel comfortable.

Cues—Teaching Tips
Keep hips square with legs strong and long front foot in a flex. Keep the spine straight.

Energetic Benefits
It brings satisfaction and courage. It inspires and deepens faith in the practice.

Physical Benefits
This is the best pose to cure sciatica problems and tone all muscles as well as nerves and tendons of the legs.

Notes:

Kurmasana—Turtle Pose

Skill: Advanced
Breath: Five to Ten
Drishti: Forward and Down
Goal: To Heal the Body
Category: General Body Stretches

Technique
From Dandasana separate the legs wide apart, bend the knees, and place the arms under the knees with the palms of the hands facing the floor and back. Bring the torso forward and lower.

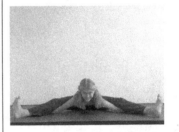

Modification
Keep the knees bended and the hands under the knees.

Cues—Teaching Tips
Keep lowering the torso until the chin touches the floor, pushing the backs of the legs down. Keep the legs strong.

Energetic Benefits
This is a sacred posture. It calms the mind and develops intuition and discernment.

Physical Benefits
It cures the body completely due to super stretches. It liberates anxiety and fears, and it tones the spine to activate the abdominal organs.

Notes:

Supta Parivrtta Garudasana— Revolved Eagle

Skill: Advanced
Breath: Five
Drishti: Sideways
Goal: To Rest with the Body in a Twist Position
Category: General Body Stretches, Twist

Technique
Lying in a supine position, bend the knees and cross one leg over the other. Try to clasp the opposite ankle behind. Rotate the body and rest. Keep arms crossed.

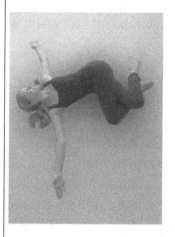

Modification
Do regular spinal twist.

Cues—Teaching Tips
The legs move toward one side while the ribs and stomach move to the other. Find the opposition.

Energetic Benefits
It invites purification and reflection on self-care. It helps to eliminate bad addictions, such as alcohol, tobacco, and recreational drugs.

Physical Benefits
It reinforces the articulations of the legs and stimulates the internal organs.

Notes:

Adho Mukha Vrksasana—Handstand

Skill: Advanced
Breath: Five to Ten
Drishti: Behind
Goal: To Develop the Body Harmoniously
Category: Inversion

Technique
From Adho Mukha Svanasana, walk the feet together toward the hands and kick one leg up, following the other. Hold them up and balance.

Modification
Practice on the wall until mastering the pose. Keep the body in the L position to bring awareness and force to the upper body.

Cues—Teaching Tips
Stay strong in the upper body and arms, with the body as straight as possible. Connect with the inner thighs.

Energetic Benefits
It delivers freedom and emancipation of life. It awakens spiritual perceptions and allows the yogi to live with abundant knowledge and wisdom.

Physical Benefits
It rejuvenates all the internal organs, strengthens the shoulders and arms, fully expands the chest, and gives inner strength.

Notes:

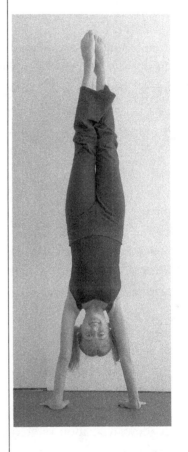

Savasana—Corpse Pose

Skill: Beginner
Breath: Three to Ten Minutes
Drishti: Eyes Closed
Goal: To Rest
Category: General Body Stretch

Technique
Lying down, separate the legs to the edge
of the mat with the feet turning out. Keep
arms long and hands facing up, with chin
toward the collarbone. Keep neck long
and eyes closed.

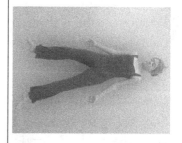

Modification
Place a blanket under the knees or a prop
in any other place.

Cues—Teaching Tips
Rest deeply, feel gratitude, and connect
with a higher source.

Energetic Benefits
It reconnects with the state of innocence
and purity of the soul.

Physical Benefits
It allows relaxation and refreshes the body.
It eliminates fatigue and relaxes the mind.

Notes: